Foreword by Professor David Ha..

Emeritus Professor of Community Paediatrics, University of Sheffield.

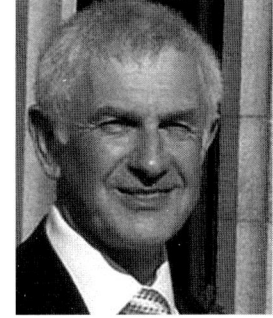

The school health service in England is almost exactly a century old, and it is worth recalling that it began because of concern about the poor health of the young men recruited for the Boer wars.

One hundred years ago, many young people suffered from under nutrition, rickets, rheumatic heart disease, impetigo and a host of other conditions which are now rarely seen in the developed world. Yet it could be argued that if one applies a holistic definition of health, young people now are no healthier than they were a century ago.

An alarmingly high proportion of our young people grow up in disrupted and unsupportive families and attend schools where bullying of all kinds is a daily occurrence, gang membership is the key to safety and mediocre education is delivered by an endless succession of supply teachers.

They live in an obesogenic environment – the lack of facilities for sport and leisure, the disappearance of family mealtimes and home cooking and the emergence of fast food all contribute. They are exposed to a constant emphasis on the desirability of early sexual activity and subtle advertising encourages the huge increase in alcohol consumption by young people. The end product of this toxic mixture is a mixture of physical and mental ill health which is outwith the experience of mainstream medical care.

It is surely no exaggeration to say that more ill health now arises in this way and more lives are blighted, than can ever be attributed to what we conventionally think of as disease. Middle-class professionals who have grown up in happy families, lived in pleasant safe neighbourhoods and attended "good" schools often have little conception of the lives of young people who lack these advantages.

Not surprisingly, school nurses who are daily confronted with these issues have been undertaking a radical rethink of their role and the extent to which they can hope to have any impact on problems that are largely social rather than medical in the origins.

A well staffed and well-trained school nursing service could make a substantial contribution to addressing at least some of the problems experienced by today's young people in schools, but inadequate funding, the endless cycle of management reorganisations and lack of agreement as to the priorities must surely limit the impact of the service as currently organised.

This wide ranging review of research on school nursing is therefore very timely – the authors have wisely concentrated on looking at the scope of the subject rather than trying to assess the quality or significance of published work. We must hope that this review will stimulate a more generous and constructive approach to the funding of research and development in this unglamorous but crucially important aspect of preventive health care.

March 2006

Acknowledgements

This work is indebted to the many school nurses who gave us their internal reports and their advice on resources and publications. Any errors or missed references are the responsibility of the authors. We hope this scope review will be the beginning of a continuously updated resource and not the "final word" on this evidence base for school nurse practice.

Contents

Introduction and overview

WHAT IS THE CHALLENGE?

School nurse practice has been difficult for most people to describe because school nurses work to a variety of contracts and in a variety of settings. They also work in the community and on school premises.

In the past decade, school nursing has developed and changed quite radically and the need to understand school nurse practice has taken on particular urgency for a range of reasons.

"The Children Act 2004 subsumes many existing planning requirements into a single children and young people's plan (CYPP) that local authorities will be required to have in place by April 2006. Authorities will work with local partners towards the recommendations and targets they set out." (www.health-for-all-children.co.uk).

In addition to impetus from the *Children Act*, NHS commissioning bodies responsible for school nurse services work to Children's Services Plans. These require inter-agency collaboration between health services, social care, youth justice, education, drug action teams, voluntary organisations, and others who provide services for children and young people. Collaboration across professional and organisational boundaries has long been a policy vision. It is now driven by legislation.

Within these large collaborative ventures at local authority level, school nurse practice is always in danger of having to struggle to make its voice heard. School nursing remains a service without legislative requirement, without a regulatory framework of its own, and without a consensus about its education and training platform. Dunnett et al (January 2005) published a helpful guidance on the demands partnership working makes on school nurses.

School nursing is the only NHS professional group whose remit is entirely, and only focused on meeting the health needs of school-aged children, young people, and their families. And yet, despite widespread innovations in practice by highly committed school nurse leaders, it remains the case that the service is still somewhat invisible.

Managers in the education sector, healthcare managers, many teachers, and many social care workers continue to misunderstand or simply not notice school nurse practice. The "invisibility" of school nursing that was documented in 1997 (DeBell and Everett) remains a problem. Furthermore, there continues to be evidence of some confusion about the range and potential overlap of work carried out by health visitors and school nurses respectively, particularly amongst specialists who design health systems.

Such confusion could well increase given that children are attending school at younger ages. In addition, the extended schools initiative will mean that many children will be in school settings for longer periods during each day. See Scotland's plans for integration of the health visitor and school nurse roles below.

"Heart of Birmingham NHS Trust is moving into corporate teams of Health Visiting and School Nursing. We see this as a fundamental change that will bring about meaningful and real partnership working. The structure will assist Practice Based Commissioning, Every Child Matters, Choosing Health as well as national strategies."
(Mary Rutledge, 5 August 2005 email message)

WHAT IS THE EVIDENCE BASE?

The purpose of this scope review is to clarify the evidence base for school nurse practice in the four countries of the United Kingdom at the outset of 2006. There have been repeated assertions that little research evidence is available about school nurse practice. This is not the case. There is a considerable evidence base for practice but it is largely focused on the activities of individual services rather than on the scope and range of school nurse practice itself. *This review extrapolates from the evidence base in order to describe the constituent elements of current practice.*

If the school nurse service were lost, there is no health professional group who could replace the work that these healthcare staff do for school age children and young people. The purpose of this scope review is to provide a much needed evidence base for managers and school nurses to use as a planning tool.

This is the first overview of research since Watters published her comprehensive literature review in 1999. Since 1999, however, there has been considerable, and sometimes radical change in school nurse practice in most parts of the United Kingdom.

The scope review presented here includes findings from government strategy and policy documents, from primary research in the field, from professional articles about service updates, and from 'grey' (unpublished) literature held by individual NHS bodies and higher education institutions.

HOW LARGE IS THE WORKFORCE?

We are frequently told that there are between 2,500 and 3,000 school nurses in the four countries of the United Kingdom but there are no national registers. We have only this entirely hypothetical figure.[1]

In 2005, the Royal College of Nursing (RCN) reported that 2,211 of its members identify "school nurse" in their job title (See Ball and Pike's 2005 survey for the RCN.)

Despite the RCN's comprehensive census survey, we still do not know the precise total for the whole of the UK workforce[2]. The RCN findings reveal that 79% of the school nurses who responded to their survey work part-time (typically 26 hours/week) and term-time only.

Furthermore, we do not know what qualifications are required for a school nurse to be able to call her/himself a "school nurse" in the 21st Century in the UK. With 11.2 million children of school age (5 – 19) in England, Wales, Scotland, and Northern Ireland, this *approximate* number of school nurses is manifestly inadequate as a resource.

●

1 Clark et al (April 2000) reported "some 200 nurses providing a service to 2000 schools with around 490,000 school children" in Wales and "not a single school nurse trained in Wales between 1995 and 2000". We do not have figures of this kind updated for Wales after 2000 nor do we have comparable figures for England or Scotland. Northern Ireland reported 93 (WTE) school nurses in 2003 (Turner and Lazenbatt 2003).

2 For example, we do not know if all Amicus-CPHVA (Community Practitioners' and Health Visitors' Association) members are also RCN members and we do not know if there are school nurses outside both professional bodies.

Despite re-orientating practice to meet targeted child health and social care needs and away from comprehensive coverage, the numbers of school nurses available to meet the diversity of children's health related need remains sufficiently low to be characterised as a human resource crisis. A skill-mix team approach is the favoured method for confronting this particular workforce planning challenge.

THIS SCOPE REVIEW

The review of the literature outlined here reveals changes in practice over the past decade as well as a diversity of settings and a diversity of professional activities in school nurse practice today.

The single most urgent research now needed is a cost and outcome measure of the effectiveness of the service. Measurement of service value against outcomes has always been a serious gap in the research about school nursing. See Cotton et al (2000) for cost analysis and Roden (1997) for the only two attempts to measure service value in this way in the UK. Also see Sheetz (2003) for a study of outcome measures for school nursing in Washington State, USA.

However, we first need to know what is expected from the service. It is this that has been unclear. Lack of clarity about service delivery, an absence of protocols with outcome measures, and poor information systems about service activities have weakened the service's ability to negotiate its terms and conditions with employers.

This scope review provides a starting point for understanding the practice of school nursing in the four countries of the UK today. It will be of considerable value if it is regularly updated. The authors invite readers to send new or missing work for inclusion in future updates.

Ⓐ Overview of research into school nurse practice

*There has been an assumption, frequently repeated, that there is very little research about school nurse practice. In fact, this is **not** the case. The problem is that studies of practice tend to be published within a narrow range of professional journals and keyword searching tends to uncover published work on children's health rather than on school nurse practice itself.*

One reason why there is a need for a scope review of school nurse practice is simply because child health actually does depend on the services that support health improvement and child well-being.

1   WHAT IS A SCOPE REVIEW?

Quite simply, a scope review is a sweep study of all the research we can find on a subject. It is not a study of the quality of the research into a subject. For example, it does not use Cochrane criteria.

What we are looking for in a scope review is the *chatter and conversation* that is going on in the field. This means that we include policy papers – those government documents that tell us what is expected of school nurses and how they are envisioned within a larger agenda for child health. But policy does not guarantee practice. On the whole, it signals directions for change in practice.

A scope review also includes descriptions of practice, whether those descriptions occur in government policy papers as untested samples of "good practice" or whether they occur in professional journals as updates on practice. This review also includes peer-reviewed research about interventions that involve school nurses where the primary focus is on child health improvement rather than primarily a focus on school nurse practice.

But a scope review also includes what we call *grey material* – this is the unpublished work that arises from student research or from internal service reviews. Many such reviews are carried out by school nurses themselves.

A scope review does not attempt to assess the quality of these individual pieces of research and reporting. In other words, we want to know about the *conversations* between practitioners and theoreticians in the field – not if the work is meeting criteria for methodological precision in research terms.

From this comprehensive overview, we then extrapolate the themes and the issues that tell us about practice. In addition, we can see from a scope review where issues are not being addressed. This matters because we need to know where there are gaps in our knowledge of school nurse practice and we also need to know where there is repetition in the studies we do have.

We also need to know why it is that school nursing is so poorly funded in the four countries of the UK. Given the sheer numbers of children, why are there so few school nurses?

A scope review of this kind also makes it possible for us to recommend where new research is needed. In other words, we do not want to keep repeating the same studies in order to find the same answers. We need to know what questions are simply not being asked.
We know, for example, that school nurse services across the UK are under-funded and short on

staff. The harsh reality is that the case for investment cannot be won simply by describing the good work that school nurses do. What we need are measures of health outcome that can be attributed to the investment itself. The economics of service delivery actually do matter. We probably have enough research now that describes the service and its practice. We need measures that tell us what the costs and the benefits of the service are.

2 WHY A SCOPE REVIEW?

In 2000, Professor Dame June Clark's project team reported on school nursing in Wales and found "*a lack of research which could constitute an evidence base for school nursing practice*" (internal document). Similarly, a taskforce for the Community Practitioners' and Health Visitors' Association (CPHVA), which was set up to study research and development in school nurse practice from 2001 to 2004, came to much the same conclusion.

This scope review was therefore designed to test these findings. If they were true, the service would be disadvantaged in finding ways to progress and to develop. In other words, assertions of value without an evidence base are always subject to disregard.

As Coote et all argued in 2004, "*There should be much more open discussion at all levels of the complex and varied roles that different kinds of evidence can play in helping to plan and implement social programmes*." (p. xiii)

We used the following key words: "school nursing", "school nurse", "school health", "school age child", "school health promotion", "child health promotion". We searched more than thirty databases. The most useful were CINAHL (Nursing and Allied Health Literature), Medline, Cochrane Library, British Nursing Index, NHS Centre for Reviews and Dissemination (York University).

Exclusions included articles in languages other than English; mainly (but not wholly) pre-1990 to 1999 publications; specific child health reports such as teenage pregnancy and childhood obesity. Though, in both these cases, we skimmed many publications for insight into school nurse practices and included a number of such reports.

We used a range of web sites but focused especially on those for the Department of Health; the Department for Education and Skills, the Northern Ireland Assembly and Executive, the Scottish Executive, the Welsh Assembly (and their predecessor departments); and also the website for Health, Social Services, and Public Safety. Other key web sites included the Royal College of Paediatrics and Child Health (RCPCH), the King's Fund, the RCN, and the CPHVA.

We had considerable difficulty locating two key American Journals, *Journal of School Nursing* (www.nasn.org/josn/journal.htm) and *Journal of School Health* (www.ashaweb.org). These are important resources for school nurse practice. At present, the British Library is the repository for hardcopies of current and back issues. On-line access requires subscription. Both journals publish excellent peer-reviewed research. We have included a small selection in the references.

The first journal for school nursing in the UK was launched in 2005, *School Health* (published in conjunction with the *Journal of Family Health*). The editors are Pat Scowen and Barbara Richardson-Todd.

We also conducted a library/hand search of journals in two university libraries (Kings College London and the University of East Anglia). The original start point for our work was 1999 but included formative work published before that date.

In conducting this scope review, some difficulties emerged that will be familiar to colleagues who have previously attempted to find an evidence base for school nurse practice. For example, keyword searching for "school nursing" repeatedly produced links to "schools of nursing". Researchers may find this insight helpful because it is indicative of the problems and human limitations that arise in any citation referral system and any database development task. It is also indicative of the way authors seek to choose keywords that will enhance the range and scope of their potential readers.

Over a period of four years from 2001 to 2005, we repeatedly tracked the field via "deep searching" and "searching to saturation". We found the following.

- There is considerable evidence of research into school nurse practice but it is not easily accessible.
- A growing variety in practice within each country in the UK and across the four countries of the UK makes it very difficult for school nurses to represent their service to stakeholders in a consistent and coherent manner.
- We now know that there is very little knowledge of the relationship between school nurse costs and the nature or extent of benefits from that investment.

3 VALUE OF AN EVIDENCE BASE FOR SCHOOL NURSE PRACTICE

A scope review: What value to school nurses?
- Evidence of the range of school nurse practice
- Evidence of "what works" in diverse locations
- Handbook for education and training
- A "start point" for understanding public health and the school age child

This scope review provides an evidence base for planning and developing services. It also provides a base on which to continue to track new and emerging research findings. Apart from the *Strategy for Practice* (DeBell and Jackson 2000), there is not a specific framework for planning school nurse services across the UK. There are, however, constituent elements of practice that all school nurses share. And each individual country (England, Scotland, Wales, and Northern Ireland) is now developing a planned "way forward".

The reality, based on this scope review, is that school nurse services are probably more diverse in their practice today than they have ever been in the past. And that, in itself, is making it difficult to represent the service to stakeholders and commissioners.

Furthermore, this report of the evidence base draws attention to the difference between government policy and its practical implementation. It is important for practitioners to recognise that policy documents are about intentions. They are not promises to deliver. *"Despite the claims made in official publications, . . . there is a gap between the rhetoric of evidence-based policy and what happens on the ground, which is a great deal more complicated."* (Coote et al, 2004, p xi)

Government policy provides a framework for planning but it is the task of the service itself to design the programmes that will match policy encouragement. A scope review of the kind presented here allows us to look at all current practice within school nursing.

During a study of North Staffordshire's school nurse service (DeBell 2000), we found that all 37 qualified school nurses in the team were regularly engaged in tracking and reading recent research and policy documents in order to inform practice. This is an indication of good professional practice in service development.

The following key texts should be in every school nurse and school nurse manager's portfolio.
- Blair, Stewart-Brown, Waterson, Crowther (2003) *Children's Public Health*. Oxford University Press: Oxford.
- Cowley (forthcoming 2006) *Community public health, policy and practice: a source book*. Elsevier: London.
- DeBell and Jackson (2000) *School Nursing within the Public Health Agenda: A Strategy for Practice*. McMillan-Scott: London.
- DeBell and Jackson (forthcoming 2007) *Public Health and the School Age Population*. Hodder Arnold: London.
- Department of Health and Department for Education and Skills (2004) *National Service Framework for Children, Young People and Maternity Services*. HMSO: Norwich.
- Department of Health (2003) *Every Child Matters*. DH: London.
- Hall and Elliman (2003, updated and reprinted June 2006) *Health for all children 4th edition*. Oxford University Press: Oxford.
- Laming (2003) *The Victoria Climbié Inquiry: Report*. HMSO: Norwich.

B The key changes in school nurse practice in the 21st century

1 THE EDUCATION – HEALTH LINK AND SOCIAL CARE

"The connection between health and education is one of the most important aspects of paediatrics. In general our understanding of disorders of learning is still rudimentary, and the problems of intellectual limitation, defective speech, inadequate reading ability, excessive clumsiness, disturbed behaviour, truancy, school phobia and delinquency create a formidable array of disability. These problems will yield only to the combined efforts of doctors, teachers, psychologists, social workers and others. Yet we have found a good deal of evidence that as yet services were not disposed to co-operate in the interests of the child." The Court Report 1976

Health

A child's physical and mental health have long been recognised as key factors in the child's ability to learn at school. However, the organisation of priorities within individual schools does not always bear this out. Berry Mayall's *Children's Health in Primary Schools* (1996) first documented the damaging split between education and health in the perception and organisation of children's schooling in England.

"Yet education also takes place at home, and health care at school. Children themselves challenge the division of lived life into private and public sectors; they take their bodies and emotions, as well as their minds, into school each day. For them the maintenance of health there is a key concern." (Mayall 1996, p 1)

The National Healthy Schools Programme

Mayall and his team drew attention to the unhealthy fabric of English schools, the poor quality food, the unhygienic toilet facilities, the endemic bullying on playgrounds. Within this actual environment, the Health Promoting Schools concept (now the National Healthy Schools Programme – NHSP) was first announced in England in December 1993 as a response to intended collaboration with the European Network of Health Promoting Schools (ENHPS). The Health Education Authority in 1997 (see Hamilton and Saunders *Summary*) published the first national evaluation of the programme's progress in England. It did not once mention school nurse services nor did it refer to any other healthcare professionals.

This absence of reference to healthcare services to schools has now begun to change. By 2005, the profile of NHSP was demonstrating active cross-departmental collaboration between the Department for Education and Skills (DfES) and the Department of Health (DH). That this link is now formalised has much to do with the initiative of school nurses in their local communities and their determination at national level to introduce school nurse skills into the health promoting schools programme. Early NHSP programmes across England and as late as 2002/03 had been notable for the widespread absence of school nurses.

School nurses and schools

Across the UK, school doctors have been quietly disappearing from school health services. It is now more common to find community paediatricians directing care for children with long-term conditions and complex health needs while school nurses self-manage school health services. The putative cost savings accrued by no longer employing school doctors has not been transferred to school nurse services.

School nurses, between 1948 and 1974, were employed directly by local education authorities. However, the history of relationship between state education and school health services has always been a matter of "invitation" to healthcare workers by schools, regardless of the employing body. School nurses are still subject to invitation by individual schools in order to work in a school. This places each school nurse in the position of "guest".

The reality, however, is that schools seriously depend upon having access to health service staff and they tend to expect a service to be provided. Independent schools generally employ a school nurse directly as do some large secondary schools in the state sector.

School head teachers, in fact, tend to be vociferous in response to any threat that they may lose their school nurse resource. It is health service staff's knowledge of child health, and their ability to win the confidence of children and their parents that is highly prized.

The reality for school nurses, nonetheless, is that they are expected to step outside traditional health service boundaries while they are simultaneously perceived to be the local voice of health service knowledge. This has always been a problematic and difficult position to occupy. The policy position, particularly for development of the NHSP, is that the health – education link is a partnership. The question is how can a 'guest' also be a partner.

School nurse initiatives

There is considerable evidence of individual demonstration projects that prove the benefit school nurse initiatives can have for child health when working closely with schools. For example, see the following, which we have randomly selected.

- Currie and Lyttle's 2004 report of school nurse work with school sex education and youth clinics in Dumfries and Galloway.
- Bekaert's 2002 study of school nurses' contribution to sexual health and contraception.
- Adelman et al reporting in 1997 on school nurse work in mental health in American schools.
- Smith's 2003 study of a school nurse pilot to deliver emergency contraception in Selby and York.
- Lister-Sharp's et al 1999 systematic reviews of health promotion in schools.
- Baptiste and Drennan's 1999 study of communication between school nurses and primary care teams.
- Bax and Whitmore's 1991 study of school nurse assessments of children at school entry.
- Bowen's 2000 study of the school nurse contribution to Middlesborough's Health Action Zone.
- Clarke's 2000 study of school nurse work with child protection.
- Croghan's 2002 study conducted with school nurses of children's access to drinking water and clean toilets at school.
- Caulfield's 1997 and Duffin's 2000 analyses of school nurses' legal position with regard to child and family consent.
- Farrell's 1998 study of asthma management in Wakefield schools.
- Laing's 1999 study of school nurse school entry interviews in Lambeth.
- Sutton's et al 2004 study of school nurse service reorganisation in Walsall.
- Wainwright's et al 2000 systematic review of the health promotion work by school nurses.

- Richardson-Todd's 2003 description of a young person's drop-in clinic in Ipswich.
- Lane and Day's 2001 study of a sexual health clinic set up by school nurses and youth workers in Sheffield.

These demonstration projects are illustrations only and we selected them at random. There are numerous such accounts. They constitute the single largest category of research from which we can extrapolate a picture of school nurse practice. However, these individual demonstration projects cannot easily be generalised across services and this produces a research challenge. At present, we do not have methods to determine the quality of these projects such that they can be transferred from one school nurse service to another.

In contrast, an effective example of nationally transferable work is the certification programme published in 2004 (Young and Arnold-Dean) for community nurses assisting in the provision of personal, social and health education (PSHE) in schools. This joint approach on behalf of the DfES, the Teenage Pregnancy Unit, and the NHSP Programme (DH) is the kind of leadership from the centre that does have the capacity to transfer policy into practice and from one service to another.

The White Paper (October 2005) on schools in England, *Higher Standards, Better Schools for All – More Choice for Parents and Pupils,* commits the government to resourcing the school nurse service in the following way. At least one full-time year-round qualified school nurse will be responsible for each cluster of primary schools and the related secondary school while taking account of health needs and school populations. The target date is 2010. This is an implicit recognition of the skill-mix team approach. And, to be achieved, it signals a senior role for qualified school nurses. What it does not do is commit resources to increasing the base number of qualified school nurses above current levels.

Social care
Similarly, the social care function has always been problematic for school nurses. Despite their work with families and in family visiting, it remains the case that school nurses do not generally play the key role in child protection. On the whole, social care remains within the domain of social services departments and health service leadership is more likely to come from health visitors than from school nurses.

This profile may well change with the introduction of the Information Sharing and Assessment initiative that is currently being rolled out across the UK. The Laming Report (2003) exposed the danger to child health of inadequate information sharing systems across the whole of the country. Notably, missing children (particularly those not at school or often missing from school) are some of the most vulnerable children and young people in all four countries of the UK. The Information Sharing and Assessment initiative is designed to ensure methods for tracking children, particularly missing children.

Enhanced attention to children who are vulnerable, on the one hand, and an increasing sophistication of knowledge about how to support parents, on the other hand, are two factors that have shifted attention away from perceiving school nurses as mainly providing services to schools.

Schools are the main community setting in which we find children but they are not the only setting. There is now an increasing recognition that school nurses work in the community and with families. The school nurse service is for children, young people, and their families. It is not simply a resource for schools.

2 PROMOTING HEALTH

The concept of health promotion

"A health promoting school is one in which all members of the school community work together to provide children and young people with integrated and positive experiences and structures, which promote and protect their health. This includes both the formal and the informal curriculum in health, the creation of a safe and healthy school environment, the provision of appropriate health services and the involvement of the family and wider community in efforts to promote health."
(World Health Organisation, 1995)

'Health promotion', 'health education', and 'public health' are often used interchangeably by practitioners. The pace of conceptual change has been radical in the last decade though 'public health' has always had an epidemiological base.

Child health promotion is not simply about individual lifestyle change. Lifestyle behaviours derive from and are a consequence of social and community cultures. Furthermore, health promotion becomes more difficult in the school age years – particularly in adolescence. As the child gains increasing independence from the family over time, the challenges in 'making a difference' actually mean that successful outcomes depend more and more on the *health promotion skills* of the school nurse workforce.

The activities identified as health promotion initiatives by school nurses are numerous but they mainly focus on individual lifestyle and health related behaviour change. It is structural change that is needed in order to promote health (see Public Health below).

The concept of 'health promotion' has become highly theorised in the past decade, mainly as a consequence of significant government investment in health promotion activities with the advent of HIV during the early 1990s.

Children and health promotion

Children themselves early identified food and exercise as the main health promoting components in their lives (see Mayall 1996). However, children have only recently begun to be asked about the features of their lives and their environment that they understand to be health promoting. Their views are an important starting point for school nurse practice.

The encouragement toward behaviours that are conducive to personal health and well-being is a complex field (see Lister-Sharp et al, 1999). Success relies on the child or family's own motivation and, particularly, success depends on the child's *social and cultural* environment. Apart from the many environmental factors (safe play areas, healthy food, access to pleasurable physical activity, safe roads, homes and housing), most health promoting behaviours are subject to personal decision-making and access to accurate information.

The interaction between individual behaviours and community level opportunities for improving health is also complex. Recent government policy has begun to recognise the important centrality of a national agenda for health promotion (*Choosing Health* 2004) as well as the role of the education sector in child health improvement (*Higher Standards, Better Schools for All*, 2005).

School nurse activities

Children and young people report a wish to have access to confidential health information, particularly about risk behaviours and emotional distress. This is a form of health promotion activity where school nurse practice plays an important role, particularly in providing drop-in clinics at school and in the community.

Immunisation against preventable infection is, of course, the starting point for both health promotion and for the public health role of school nursing. But school nurses report that they are also working in health promotion activities across all contemporary issues from dental caries to sun protection.

In some parts of the UK, school nurses have acquired postgraduate qualifications in health promotion. There are good arguments for including a team member with this kind of higher level qualification as a resource within each school nurse team.

The integration of school nurses into the PSHE (personal, social and health education) and Sex Education curricula in schools (the health education focus) as well as integration with the NHSP is likely to bring coherence to a field that otherwise can become an accident of individual school nurse "interest".

Note that "good" practice in school nursing often goes unrecorded and is thereby not reported outside the locality in which it is located. Not every effective innovation is studied and/or published.

Accuracy, appropriacy, and good timing are the three factors that Hall and Elliman (2003) identify as key to good health promotion. This implies that school nurses, in developing their health promoting role, need to be cognisant of age appropriate interventions as well as precisely accurate about the health information that children receive. Furthermore, health promotion is a matter of staged repetition. For example, sexual health promotion needs to be iterative and age appropriate. It also needs to be context specific. This means that location and timing of service delivery is as important for effectiveness as is the content.

Furthermore, parental support programmes are a form of health promotion and our knowledge about which approaches are most effective in this field is increasing exponentially.

Child health & social care issues for the UK in the 21st century
- Child and adolescent mental health needs
- Long-term conditions and complex health needs
- Injuries (accidental and non-accidental)
- Vulnerability and child protection
- Sexual health needs

- Childhood obesity (nutrition and exercise)
- Risk behaviours

3 CHILD AND ADOLESCENT MENTAL HEALTH (CAMHS)

Overview

The estimates for numbers of children who experience mental health problems at some point during their school age years vary between 10% (National Audit Office) and 20% (Young Minds) of the total school age population. *This is the largest single source of health need amongst school-aged children and young people in the UK*. But these figures refer to mental health distress, not to mental disorders, which are rare amongst school-aged children.

A child in primary school may well describe stress or anxiety in terms of a tummy or headache or may claim physical illness without apparent physical cause. Similarly, both enuresis and encopresis can be indications of emotional distress. School nurses are historically a key resource for teachers and parents in cases where early assessment and appropriate referral for specialist assistance is needed.

Assessing mental health

Recognising mental distress, quite apart from assessing how and when to help these children and young people, is fraught with difficulty. At school, parents or school staff may notice mood change, withdrawal or aggression, age-inappropriate behaviours, changes in eating or sleeping habits, irritability, inability to concentrate, clumsiness or tendencies to become accident prone, aggression and/or bullying, self-harm, unexplained accidents or injury. Any of these can indicate emotional distress.

Large secondary schools have more difficulty monitoring individual child emotional needs of this kind than do, for example, small primary schools. It is also the case that emotional problems manifest differently in different age groups (the young child, the middle school years, and the adolescent). The implications for school nurse practice therefore suggest a need for different skills to meet the needs of each age group.

School nurse practice

Repetition in the evidence base tells us that the school nurse has often been a first port of call for emotional problems. In our research in 1996 (DeBell and Everett 1997), Norfolk school nurses repeatedly told us that "counselling children and parents" was the task they were most often called upon to do and the task they found most demanding.

Since 1996, there has been significant (though not sufficient) progress in both the skills of recognition and the provision of services for children and young people with mental health problems but those skills and knowledge are not systematically included in all school nurse development programmes.

Child and adolescent mental health is an area in which expectations about school nurse delivery are only sporadically matched with good quality education and training for school nurses.

What then is the school nurse responsibility and how is it reflected in school nurse practice? In terms of the Health Advisory Service (HAS 1995) Tier 1 to 4[3] assessment profiles, school nurses have a Tier 1 referral function. In some school nurse services, individual staff have gone further and have allocated individual school nurses the training and resources they need in order to develop specialist skills in mental health support for children and young people at Tier 2 (e.g., see Bath & North East Somerset PCT).

But the reference to "counselling" by Norfolk school nurses in 1996 has always been and continues to be problematic, if not worrying. The term "counselling", when used by school nurses, tends to refer to advice – to the child, the parent, or the teacher. In effect, *where this is offered without professional training*, the school nurse plays the same informal role as does any good 'befriender'.

In some cases, the growing sophistication of expertise about parenting support has become an important resource for school nurses working with child mental health problems. But that too requires a good education and training base. Yet again, work in parenting support requires considerable formal training. Both "counselling" and parenting support skills demand focused and well-resourced training if school nurses are to be effective as well as responsible practitioners.

Health and education perspectives

Where a teacher observes "disruptive behaviour" a school nurse is likely to observe "mental or emotional distress". Education professionals refer to mental health problems as "emotional and behavioural" problems. Health professionals refer to child and adolescent "mental health problems". Language matters in this field, not least because it is a key to inter-professional communication.

Where emotional and behavioural problems are concerned, school nurse practice is about an ability to differentiate between normative (daily upsets) and non-normative stress (e.g., arising from traumatic or unusual experiences – illness, bereavement, abuse, family breakdown). See Lau (2002).

Many writers refer to the school nurse as "ideally placed" (Lightfoot and Bines 2000), "pivotal" (Leighton 2003), "well placed" (Thompson et al 2003) to support anxious and stressed children. However, such assertions presume school nurses are "available" when needed. The reality, of course, is that some schools "see" a school nurse only once or twice each term.

In addition, a few school nurses have been provided with exceptionally sophisticated training in order to work in the CAMHS field but most have not.

The general profile of practice suggests that school nurses need training and development as well as referral skills in order to assess appropriately when responding to the mental health needs of children and young people. Clark et al (2003) reported school nurse staff feeling "overwhelmed" by the complex mental health problems of some children. Leighton's (2003) research confirmed that further training is needed for school nurses to feel confident about dealing with these issues. And this feeling of "professional inadequacy" is echoed by Lightfoot and Bines (2000)[4]. Yet, the *School Nurse Development Resource Pack* (Department of Health 2001) asserts that promoting good mental health is a core component of the school nurse's role.

3 Despite critiques of the Tier 1, 2, 3, 4 model, we use it here for ease of reference.

4 Jewell C. (2004).

4 LONG-TERM CONDITIONS AND COMPLEX HEALTH NEEDS

"As numbers of children with conditions that require medical attention during school hours grow, so do the numbers of teachers who express their inadequacy. Teachers report an inability to cope because they do not understand medical conditions and feel unprepared to handle emergencies." (Siminerio and Koerbel, 2000)

This familiar observation raises two questions: the role of teachers in healthcare and the changing profiles of child health needs (e.g., the rise in conditions such as asthma and diabetes, the mainstreaming agenda in education, and the child's right to attend school and the child's right to receive appropriate healthcare).

Teachers are understandably anxious about providing direct care without appropriate training. Furthermore, the teachers' unions have repeatedly urged their members not to administer medication to school children. At the same time, see *Access to Education for Children and Young People with Medical Needs* (2001), *Supporting Pupils with Medical Needs* (1997) and *Managing Medicines in Schools and Early Years Settings* (2005). Hall and Elliman (2003) suggest that many of these care and medication issues can be sensibly managed via school nurses helping teachers with basic training and, in some cases, by health staff negotiating adjustments in the timing for administering medication (i.e., adjustments that avoid the school day).

Research findings over the years have also repeatedly drawn attention to the difficulties teachers have in understanding nurse confidentiality agreements with children and young people. Teachers have frequently reported that they wish school nurses to be more forthcoming about children – e.g., anxieties about "keeping secrets" (see Mukherjee et al, 2002). These are inter-professional communication issues (see Lightfoot and Bines, 2000) that deserve time and attention.

"The big public health question is how do you get maximum health gain, within limited resources, for this group of children and their families?" (Dr Simon Lenton, community paediatrician, email message 15 December 2005).

The resource issue is paramount in determining direction of service generally but it is particularly challenging in circumstances where school age children and young people have long-term conditions and complex health needs. There are current staff shortages across the UK in the following areas: social work staff; school nurses; public health nurses and health visitors; paediatricians; child and adolescent mental health services staff; therapists; orthoptists. Both community health services and children's services have always been under-resourced – an historic issue that beleaguers the whole issue of school nurse practice development.

And children who have particularly special needs during their school years require particularly special assistance from healthcare staff.

5 VULNERABLE CHILDREN AND YOUNG PEOPLE

"Growing Support"(2002), a Scottish review of multi-agency support provided for vulnerable families with very young children, found a broad consensus across professional and support agencies about the factors that make children and families more likely to be vulnerable. There was less agreement about the respective agencies' responsibilities to intervene." (Hall and Elliman 2003, p 21-22)

In other words, it is not difficult to explain the causes or describe the circumstances of vulnerability but the real challenge is agreeing ways to reverse vulnerability. This is the use that "good practice" examples are put to but they do not usually describe the criteria that underlie the assessment of "good practice".

Scotland, for example, has reported (2004h) that "*much health care was reactive, and preventative work took little account of the difficulties that vulnerable families may have in following the comprehensive and sensible advice offered*" (7.16). The Scottish recommendation is that "*A greater focus on health promotion and direct work with parents rather than routine health surveillance would better meet the needs of vulnerable families*".

Vulnerability is not a simple concept. On the whole, it tends to refer to children who are in need of additional care and attention because of the circumstances of their lives.

- Children not at school, including those excluded or truanting
- Children in secure or special residential care with associated educational provision
- Children in hospital or residential care
- Children looked after by local authorities
- Children living with mobile families, including refugees and asylum seekers
- Children living with informal carers
- Homeless young people
- Children acting as carers
- Children in poverty

Following the *Laming Report* (2003), the concept of vulnerability has been significantly widened in order to include children and young people who are "missing" in the sense that they are not necessarily known to public services. These include the children of mobile or loosely organised family units, the children of refugees and asylum seekers, and children who are homeless. A number of models have been derived to pictorially represent gradations of vulnerability (see Hall and Elliman 2003, p 20). Also, see below a model based on analysis of Newham Borough Council, which has a very high proportion of children and young people as percentage of population, many of whom are "vulnerable".

Figure 1 Needs distribution model reflecting Newham child population[5]

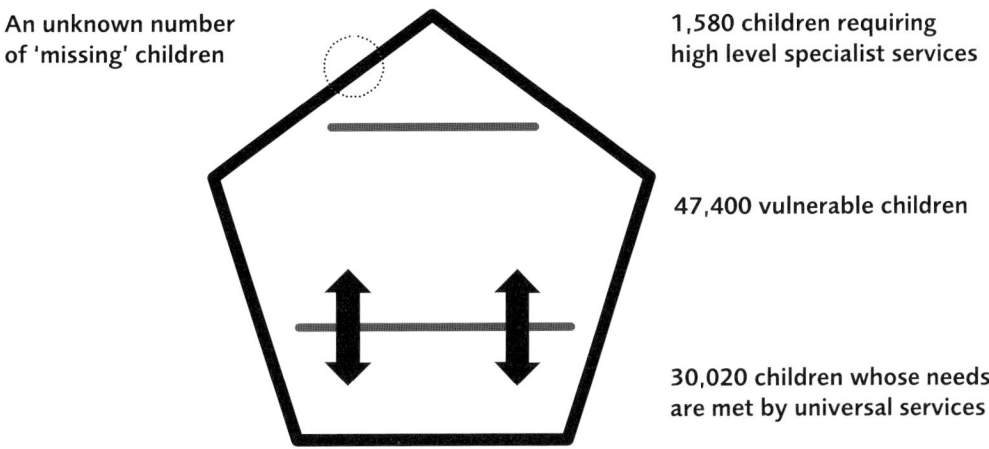

An unknown number
of 'missing' children

1,580 children requiring
high level specialist services

47,400 vulnerable children

30,020 children whose needs
are met by universal services

Figure 2 Standard needs distribution model

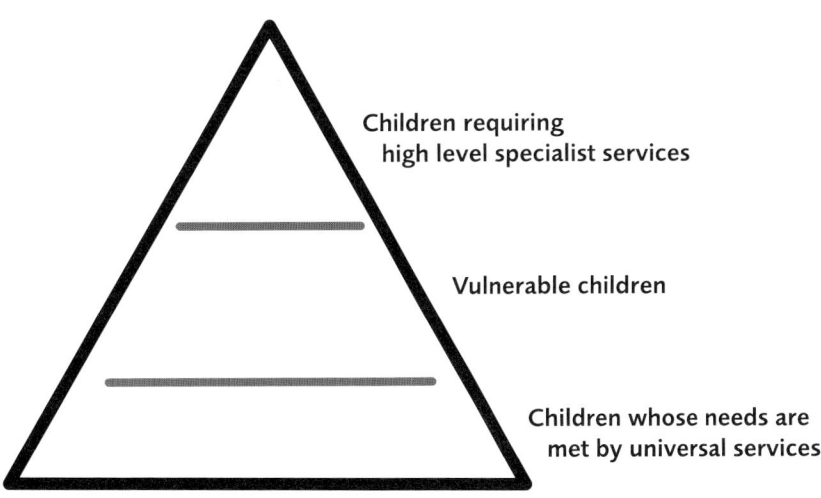

Children requiring
high level specialist services

Vulnerable children

Children whose needs are
met by universal services

The above modelling is an example of how a local authority can analyse its child population for planning purposes in order to concentrate services more effectively.

The Information Sharing and Assessment (ISA) initiative designed to protect vulnerable children is likely to become an important feature of school nurse practice. However, there is as yet no systematic plan to deliver the information technology resources that school nurses need for this work. One of the key findings in Northern Ireland (Turner and Lazenbatt 2003) referred to the failure to provide community nurses with personal computers – a basic tool for both the public health role and the ISA work required of school nurses.

5 Reproduced and amended from McKay I. *The Information, referral and tracking (IRT) project: issues for implementation in the London Borough of Newham*. Paper 1PrD, June 2003:7 and Paper 2 PrD, October 2003:3 (amended).

C School nursing – what have we learned?

1 THE EVIDENCE WE HAVE

The key changes in school nurse practice in the UK in the 21st century
- Paradigmatic shift from medical to social model of child health
- Focus on public health practice
- Increasing specialisation of skills
- Team organisation and skill-mix
- Leadership for school age child and family health improvement

Practice

In the past decade, there has been a paradigm shift in school nurse practice from a medical model to a social model of working. In terms of practice, this means that school nurses no longer work alone and they no longer focus their primary attention on weighing, measuring, and checking children for defects or abnormalities. Nor do they attempt to "see" every child. Theoretically, the approach is to target scarce resource on those children and young people most in need and to provide services to groups of children. The favoured approach is to work in teams alongside other education and social care practitioners as well as with community development workers and voluntary agencies.

The approach now is preventive and collaborative rather than mainly clinical in focus and, in theory, is no longer professionally isolated – in most cases. Furthermore, government policy is ahead of practice. Since 1999, school nurse practice has been highlighted as an area for development and change.

"We need to develop the public health role of the school nurse too, building on the opportunities their contact with children and young people provide. We want them to draw on their nursing knowledge and pastoral care experience to support policies such as the healthy schools initiative. We want them to help young people make healthy lifestyle choices, to reduce risk-taking behaviour and to focus on issues such as teenage parenthood. They will need to continue to work in teams in partnership with teachers, health visitors and others to provide an integrated programme of support and health promotion." (*Making a Difference* 1999)

Policy

Yet, at the same time, government policy about school nurse development remains rhetorical in the sense that resources have not followed the activities envisioned for practice (see also *Saving Lives* 1999, *Liberating the Talents* 2003, *Chief Nursing Officer's Review* 2004).

The four categories of specialisation that were agreed by school nurses from England, Scotland, Wales, and Northern Ireland during 1999 (DeBell and Jackson 2000) remain the favoured method of organising advanced training and service delivery in most parts of the UK:

- Promoting healthy lifestyles and healthy schools
- Child and adolescent mental health
- Long-term conditions[6] and complex health care needs in children and young people
- Vulnerable children and young people.

6 The original publication (2000) used the term "chronic". Consultation with parents has resulted in an important change in terminology – now "long-term conditions".

Evidence

There is a plethora of studies about individual school nurse practice across all four of these areas of activity. And there is emerging evidence that individual school nurses are specialising in their practice where they can (e.g., sexual health, child and adolescent mental health, asthma, epilepsy, diabetes, health promotion, public health profiling).

However, the research base is mainly dominated by reports of demonstration projects. The problem with this small-scale case study reporting approach is that individual innovations ("good practice") are spread across the country, are not systematically shared between NHS trusts for planning purposes, and they reinforce the view that school nurse teams work in isolation from each other. Such demonstration projects are informative as research initiatives but they are not necessarily generalisable.

Small-scale studies and evaluations of local innovations dominate the published research, as well as the 'grey' literature. This work boosts morale amongst school nurses but it has a limiting effect on development because it does not allow us to conduct analyses that compare service interventions for quality. There is need for large scale and comparative studies across the four countries of the UK.

Dissemination activities

The response of the workforce to more than a decade of under-investment has also manifested itself in a desire to prove the value of the service by disseminating examples of innovation and change. This is a valuable and important part of the development trajectory. Yet, however important this is, dissemination of innovation projects is not sufficient on its own.

School nurses are the only dedicated generic health workers for school-aged children and young people in the community. Until school nursing is studied as a national workforce, the work of these healthcare practitioners will continue to be misunderstood, invisible, and under-resourced.

School nurses – what have we learned?
- Trusted by children and young people
- Knowledgeable
- Caring
- Skilled in working with children, young people, and their families
- Have access to settings where children and young people gather

Innovation

Furthermore, patterns of effective innovation over the past decade suggest that school nurse leaders tend to emerge naturally out of frontline practice and then to move into generic management posts in the health service and thus away from the frontline. This produces a cycle of resource loss and a repetitiveness of re-invention.

The issues that arise from the findings of this scope review are linked.

- What education and training provision is appropriate for meeting the increased skills base that is needed for school nurses so that they can address the health needs of school age children and young people in the 21st century?
- What investment is required to ensure the provision of a dedicated health resource for school-aged children and young people?
- What workforce capacity is needed in order to operate effectively in what is a shift from a curative/medicine-based focus to a health promotion and public health based focus?
- There is need to establish a register of school nurse services within each of the four countries of the United Kingdom and a formal method to ensure these nurses can share what they believe is effective in their practice.
- What are the likely associations that the name "school nurse" itself has in the public and professional imagination?
- There is need for a correlation between the numbers in any school nurse workforce and local child deprivation levels.
- School nurses need appropriate tools for their work – personal computers are a priority for any professional with a public health practice brief.

2 UNDERSTANDING PUBLIC HEALTH PRACTICE AND THE SCHOOL AGE CHILD

"There is a consensus that school nurses have a public health role, but not clarity on what that really means." (Webster 1999, p 4)

Current thinking now asserts that school nurses cannot plan effective service delivery without assessing and prioritising local health needs. This is the public health dimension. School nurses in some parts of the UK have been developing skills in individual school profiling since the mid-1990s. In a few cases, they have developed skills in epidemiology for this purpose with assistance from their directors of public health (e.g., Huddersfield).

The public health function in nursing is about making assessments of care for children based on an understanding of the local community and the environment in which the child lives. This is about a way of "seeing" health problems.

"Essentially public health is a distinctive way of seeing health problems: public health nurses and doctors ask different questions about their practice, requiring them to look beyond individuals to populations, such as:
- Why is this happening?
- How often?
- What is the social context?
- Who else should be involved?
- What works and what doesn't?

They also make different connections: between one individual and another, between individuals and communities, between individuals and social structures, between the stories that people tell them and the epidemiological evidence, between health services and other agencies, between medical and social models of health and

between health and social policies. Public health nurses, moreover, tend to have a commitment to a set of values based on equity, justice and work for social change at local and national levels." (Billingham, 1997, p 271)

The contention that school nurse practice is a public health role is not a new insight. In 1908, Lina Rogers described an entirely familiar approach to the development of school nursing. Here she tells us how and why (in 1903) she created a school nurse service in New York City. The service began as an observation about exceptionally high rates of school exclusion and a determination to address this by means of health care support.

"After a month's experimental work, made by one nurse as a demonstration, the results were considered so satisfactory that twelve nurses were appointed, and following the report of this month's work with twelve nurses in forty-eight schools (four schools for each nurse), the Board of Health considered that the work . . . had fully demonstrated its practical value as a supplement to the medical inspectors. It was seen that the work of the nurses connected the efforts of the Department of Health with the homes of the children, thus supplying the link needed to complete the chain . . ." (Rogers, 1908, p 966)

Again, in 1941, the subject of school nurse practice as a public health role was revisited.

"We called our enterprise "public health nursing". Our basic idea was that the nurse's peculiar introduction to the patient and her organic relationship with the neighbourhood should constitute the starting point for a universal service to the region. Our purpose was in no sense to establish an isolated undertaking. We planned to utilize, as well as to be implemented by, all agencies and groups of whatever creed which were working for social betterment, private as well as municipal. Our scheme was to be motivated by a vital sense of the interrelation of all these forces. For this reason we consider ourselves best described by the term 'public health nurses'. (Wales, 1941, p xi)

In both of these reports, we see the constituent elements of the public health role in contemporary school nurse practice in the UK today: the child in its family environment and at school; the child within its neighbourhood; the co-ordination of services across agencies; the pressure to achieve equity; the broader concept of health as a consequence of cultural and economic factors.

Furthermore, Grant, writing in 1942, might well have been speaking to those who wrote *Choosing Health* in 2005.

"The school health service should be of such educational value that children learn how to protect their health, to secure medical care when it is needed, and to accept reasonable responsibility for their own health and that of others. Moreover, the parents should be taught how to give their children the care necessary to promote health and maintain efficiency and happiness." (Grant, p 194-195)

3 SCHOOL NURSES – THE WORK THEY DO

We have already called attention to the increasing diversity and range of work carried out by school nurses in the four countries of the UK. Scotland (see below) has determined to formalise this in terms of (1) a core programme; (2) core + structured additional support; (3) core + intensive inter-agency support.

The National Service Framework (2004) and Hall and Elliman (2003) have provided a particularly clear framework for the core work of school nurse practice.

At the same time, the settings in which school nurse practice takes place have helpfully moved out of the tight constraints of school premises alone.

School nurses – the work they do
- Classroom advice and resource to teachers
- Drop-in centres and clinics
- Work with community groups
- Work with families
- Access to other health and social care workers
- School entry health reviews
- Immunisation coordinators

However, there still remains a tendency amongst many school nurses to target their service to meet the needs of their individual clients (individual schools or families) *without* undertaking a systematic analysis of population level needs within the communities they serve. There is also still very little evidence of consultation with children and young people about their own views of the health services they need and will want to use. (See Article 12 of the *UN Convention on the Rights of the Child* 1989.)

And, despite the inadequacy of the measure, it is still common for school nurses to talk about their work in terms of caseload size rather than social and health deprivation levels. Caseload is an inadequate measure for a service that no longer delivers the same provision to every child.

Furthermore, 'caseload' generally refers to the number of schools plus the numbers of children as a total of the children on roll. This implies that a school nurse must attend equally to *all* these schools and *all* these children.

There is urgent need for a resource allocation formula that makes sense, for example, in terms of child deprivation levels and community level health need profiles. The caseload measure has the effect of exacerbating an already substantial inequity of resource allocation.

See public health discussion above and health inequalities below.

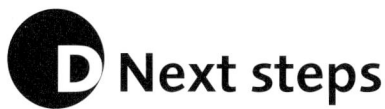 Next steps

1 THE HEALTH INEQUALITIES AGENDA

"Reducing inequalities is a definable and measurable aim that involves a range of legislative and policy initiatives, such as increased investment in education, financial benefits, help for parents who experience conflicts between child care and the need to work, pre-school provision, support for families of children with special needs, etc. This policy goal, which we support, requires a refocusing of child health services" (Hall and Elliman, 2003, p. 13).

Perhaps the greatest research advances for a social model of healthcare in the last decade have been those that help to explain the health inequalities profiles that we find across all four countries of the UK. Much of this work derives from research momentum at international level that seeks to understand the consequences for child health of health inequalities.

The accidents of birth – who are the child's parents/carers; what is their income; what is the parental/carer educational achievement level; where does the child live? These are the kinds of factors that most radically affect health profiles. These are also the key issues for public health assessments that can guide practitioners in how to target the school nurse resource most effectively.

2 THE SHAPE OF THE NEW SCHOOL NURSE TEAMS

"We travelled hard, but it seemed that every time we were beginning to form up in teams we would be reorganised, and later I was to learn in life that we tend to meet every situation by reorganising, and a wonderful method it can be for creating the illusion of progress while producing confusion, inefficiency and demoralisation." (Petronius, Governor of Bithynia, 65 BC)[7]

As late as the end of the 20th century, school nurses in most parts of the UK were working independently and alone with sole responsibility for an assigned number of named schools. The diversity of management and accountability models across England, for example, suggested little agreement about how to manage these school nurses. In fact, despite diverse models, most school nurses were directly managed by health visitors and worked virtually as assistants to school doctors.

At the same time, school nurse managers in some geographic areas (e.g., Jackson at Optimum Health Services NHS Trust in South London, Bagnall for the Queen's Nursing Institure, the school nurses within a Norfolk community trust led by Branson and Reading) were arguing a move toward skill-mix teams to be led by school nurse managers. That principle is now the dominant organising model for school nurse services across all four countries. The main exceptions are those school nurses who work independently because they are in highly remote rural areas or they work in the independent sector.

However, no sooner had the skill-mix principle been embraced than national health services were re-organised from the centre with primary care assuming a major commissioning role. One immediate consequence was the loss of the large community health trusts. Thus many of the larger clusters of school nurses were broken into smaller managed groups. In one sense, boundary changes have been (and continue to be) a feature of school nurse organisation

7 Nash et al (1985).

challenge since transfer of the service out of local authority responsibility following the NHS Reorganisation Act 1973.

For the foreseeable future, the management of school nursing will remain the responsibility of primary care commissioning bodies but with variations about how this works in each of the four countries.

Local authority targets

In a sense, we are returning to the principles of the pre-1973 approach to organisation via local authority level responsibility for children's services. The new children's trusts, though virtual in one sense, are the means whereby services will be integrated and assessed for effectiveness. And the children and young people's plans (CYPP) from April 2006 will be implemented from local authority level and they will require outcome targets.

What does this mean for frontline workers such as school nurses? Effectively, it has no immediate consequence for development of the core school nurse service and its practice. But, strategically, it is a move that does challenge school nurses to clarify their working practices and to do so in terms of the outcomes they intend to achieve.

Skill-mix

Skill-mix is an efficiency measure in this agenda. In other words, the thinking runs along the following lines. The most highly trained school nurses should be managing a planned service in which they delegate to appropriate colleagues those areas of work that require specific skills. Managing immunisation programmes is one example. Managing and delegating the tasks of school entry health reviews is another. Information management is yet another. The danger, of course, is that skill-mix can be mistaken for grade-mix. Ideally, skill-mix should include multi-professional staff (e.g., social care workers, mental health workers, health promotion specialists and people with epidemiological skills). This would mean a critical shift away from the generalist school nurse role of the past. (See Turner and Lazenbatt, 2003, p 24.)

The principle behind skill-mix teams also presumes access to appropriate education and training for specialist school nurse practitioners. This basic requirement is being achieved in certain parts of the UK – mainly in locations such as the Midlands where school nurses have easy access to clusters of higher education institutions.

A second principle behind skill-mix teams also presumes that team leaders can and will play strategic roles in service design and will manage the interface with children's trusts and with the NHSP.

However, there is still no regulatory framework specific to school nursing. This inhibits the service in gaining consistency in education and training. The profession is not yet in control of the preparation of its own practitioners.

3 DEVOLUTION: VIEWS FROM SCOTLAND, WALES AND NORTHERN IRELAND

Each of the four countries now has a Children's Commissioner. In all four cases, these post holders have committed themselves to child and family involvement in decision making about services and have committed themselves to the involvement of nurses in priority setting. These posts are designed to function as independent advocates for children as well as a link across all services and between children and government. These children's commissioners have a particular responsibility for ensuring children's rights.

Since 1999, responsibility for health and social care has been devolved from Westminster Parliament to departments in each of the four countries. Only legislation, standards and international treaties, such as *The Children Act* 2004, the *National Service Framework for Children* 2004, and the *UN Convention on the Rights of the Child* 1989, apply across the UK. However, there is continuous articulation of policy between the four countries (e.g., the findings and actions that have followed on from the *Laming Report* 2003).

Where practice is concerned, differences in approach to school nurse development are emerging in each of the four countries. All are based on a public health approach to practice. All imply an understanding of the importance of school nurse practice within community nursing and as actors in the portfolio of services for children and young people of school age.

The following are profiles of national level planning in Scotland, Wales and Northern Ireland.

SCOTLAND

Scotland has been far more radical than England, Wales, or Northern Ireland in its proposals for school nurse practice development. A review in 2001 (Scottish Executive 2001d) proposed the development of a public health nursing role that incorporates health visiting and school nursing. Furthermore, Scotland has been piloting the Family Health Nurse concept (WHO 2000a) – "family-focused community nursing and midwifery programmes and services" (p 2).

The Cabinet Delivery Group on Children and Young People, including the First Minister and Ministers with responsibility for health, education, justice, communities and finance as well as workforce development, has developed a systematic consultation based on Hall and Elliman 2003. The Group refers to this as "Hall 4".

Summary point 11: "*The national school nursing framework broadens the role of school nursing to include developing health needs assessment for schools, more active involvement in health promotion and supporting schools with the change required to enable mainstreaming of children who require additional support for learning. By 2007, all schools will be expected to become Integrated Community Schools and school nurses will be an integral part of the multi-disciplinary team. The school nursing framework signalled a need for additional investment to increase the number of staff to meet these new demands.*"

And in Summary point 10: "*The reduction in the number of routine contacts and developmental checks by public health nurses should enable redirection of public health nursing to additional or intensive support for vulnerable children and families.*"

Scotland has been carrying out a cross-agency, whole nation consultation exercise with continuous feedback from professional groups (*Health for all children 4: Guidance on Implementation in Scotland* 2005). Its position is that first responsibility lies with parents and this refers to all those with parental responsibility, including carers (see 1.7 and 1.9). Furthermore, its planning is based on health promotion and an integrated approach to service delivery.

For the first time, recommendations are for children's care from birth to adolescence (1.17).

Scotland has specified a school nurse framework and identified Health Boards as responsible for implementation. The school nursing framework:

- Delivering the core programme of Hall 4
- Proactive in assessing and meeting the health needs of each school
- Promoting healthy lifestyles and healthy schools[8]
- Supporting children with chronic (sic)[9] and complex health needs
- Supporting vulnerable children and young people.

This framework matches the programme identified in DeBell and Jackson (2000).

Furthermore, the framework places school nurse practice in diverse settings and delivery is both during and out of term time. It includes skills in community practice and school profiling with particular attention to the identification of vulnerable children. Furthermore, the guidance includes independent schools.

School nursing is positioned within the primary care setting and *the intention is to develop new models of community based nursing based on public health nursing. The plan is to bring together health visiting and school nursing* (see 2.7). 100% of 4 year olds and 85% of 3 year olds in Scotland are in some form of pre-school education environment.

Scotland's programme of development is particularly proactive and it is consistent with World Health Organisation models based on development of Community Health Partnerships.

Furthermore, Scotland addresses the tasks involved in working with families who do not trust the statutory services (3.9) and refers to need for supervision to be available to frontline staff. This is consistent with the recommendations of the *Laming Report* 2003.

Scotland is also working on a school health profiling tool (3.15) in order to inform the sctivities of the school nursing service within each school.

"The role of the school nursing service will move away from a focus on routine surveillance, towards a combination of school population-focused health improvement, and addressing the individual health needs of vulnerable children." (3.15)

". . .there should be a named nurse for each school, with access to a wider team of health support such as community children's nurses, paediatricians and therapists." (3.16)

The guidance also addresses specific actions that are measurable.

8 Scotland uses three strands – food, physical activity, and mental wellbeing.

9 See Footnote 4.

- Nutrition (free fruit schemes, breakfast clubs, fruit and salad bars and healthy tuck shops in schools)
- Physical activity measures
- Oral health measures (registration with a dentist, foods, tooth brushing skills)
- Unintentional injury monitoring
- Sexual health
- Smoking
- Drugs and alcohol.

> **"The Scottish Framework for Nursing in Schools highlights the role of school nurses in supporting the multi-agency effort required to promote healthy attitudes to drugs and alcohol, through the provision of advice and support to teachers, children and young people, and their families. School nurses also provide an important link between NHS primary care services, schools, local DAATs and specialist addiction services."** (3.51)

Information collection and sharing

The Parent Held Child Health Report (PHCHR) was introduced a decade ago and this is now recommended for adoption as the basis for recording information on child health (8.16). At present, the form of the PHCHR tends to vary in each local Health Board system. A United Kingdom working group has reviewed and revised the PHCHR as a consequence of recommendations from Hall and Elliman 2003.

Using a Parent Held Child Record, Scotland has committed itself to developing integrated care pathways to include health, education and social services (5.24 – 5.26). The *Integrated Assessment Framework (Scotland* forthcoming*)* includes information sharing – a common frame of reference rather than multiple sets of data in the hands of diverse organisations and professional groups. At a national level, a common data set would mean that the profile and detail follow the child from school to school and from geographic area to geographic area. This is consistent with the *Information Sharing and Assessment* tool 2005.

The Scottish Executive has established a Maternal and Child Health Information Strategy Group (MCHISG) to develop an integrated system using electronic technology. This will also support public health data collection as well as child health needs. A strategy for *eCare* pilots has been developed.

The Scottish experience is an example of national level comprehensive focus on child health. It is particularly notable for its consultative and comprehensive approach to child health and its explicit commitment to ensuring the improvement of child health by refocusing services.

WALES

Wales, in 2000, was the first of the four countries to appoint a Children's Commissioner. It has also set up a national Children's and Young People's Assembly, known as *Funky Dragon*. In addition, local authorities have set up forums and all schools have school councils.

The office of the Commissioner was initially established as an outcome of Part V of the Care Standards Act 2000 to reflect recommendations in the Waterhouse report (2000) *Lost in Care:*

the Report of the Tribunal of Inquiry into the abuse of children in care in the former county council areas of Gwynedd and Clwyd since 1974. The office had its original roots in the social care sector but now works closely with health.

The Welsh children's strategy has been in place since 2001 and all 22 local authorities have developed formal partnership arrangements with the health service and voluntary organisations. Free school breakfasts in subscribing primary schools are also now in place. The Welsh Assembly Government is piloting a foundation phase for children between 3 and 7 years old to assist in transition from home to school.

Wales has premised its children's health agenda on two driving issues: child poverty and children's rights. As an extension of this starting point, Wales has prioritised parenting support (*Parenting Action Plan* 2005) and has specifically identified issues around mental health and targeted attention to health surveillance of child development delay.

In addition, the Welsh approach is closely aligned with guidance on safeguarding children (2000) via the Local Safeguarding Children Board (LSCB) and ensuring children's welfare. The arrangements for information sharing in Wales are set out in regulatory directions by the Assembly Government following its devolved powers for secondary legislation.

Dame Professor June Clark's research team produced the first comprehensive analysis of school nurse practice in Wales (2000). We are not aware of a follow-up study. Her team accurately reported a key structural problem facing school nursing at that point.

"There is a conflict between current emphasis on public health and the policy of a 'primary care led NHS'. The narrow definition of primary care as services provided by the contractor professions, and in particular the organisational arrangements which were developed to support GP fundholding, have inhibited the development of other primary health care services such as school health services and workplace and other community based initiatives. . ." (Clark et al, April 2000, p. 4).

'Fundholding' has since been replaced with a commissioning model. The question is whether or not primary care commissioning has been able to restore development of community based services such as school nursing. There is also a persistent question across the whole of the UK about the difficulties of building community based programmes around primary care practice populations.

Clark concluded that school nursing in Wales, like health visiting and district nursing, is under-developed, under managed and under resourced. Her team recommended pilot sites for seconding school nurses to Local Health Groups (LHGs). Their work should include health needs assessment and population profiling.

There is need for a national study of practice comparisons across all four countries. There is also need for a follow-up to the Clark report for Wales.

NORTHERN IRELAND

Northern Ireland's Children's Commissioner is fully independent of government. *"He has a clear rights framework with strong investigatory powers and he can bring or intervene in legal proceedings on behalf of a child"*. (Comment 2005 by the National Society for the Prevention of Cruelty to Children – NSPCC).

Northern Ireland's Department of Health, Social Services and Public Safety (DHSSPS) published its *Position Paper* (November 2003) on community nursing in Northern Ireland based on widespread consultation and the work of Turner and Lazenbatt (July 2003). Its position is that *"everyone working in primary and community health and social care"* will *"think first of what the person or community needs, and then what we, together, can do about it. Thus, titles become less important and patient journeys become more important"* (p 5).

Like Scotland, Northern Ireland began implementing change in line with "Hall 4" recommendations (Hall and Elliman 2003) from April 2004. Unlike Scotland, Northern Ireland will not be changing existing community nursing titles, including school nursing. However, the thrust of planning is firmly based on a public health model as in Scotland (see Scottish Executive 2001c) and is designed to *"provide advanced generalist services, in teams, with a range of skills"* (*Position Paper* p 5). The trajectory is a twenty-year regional strategy for health and wellbeing.

The DHSSPS has funded a number of pilot projects to test new models of service delivery in different parts of NI (*Investing for Health* 2000). These are being evaluated before transfer to other primary care settings across the country. The aim is to align the community nursing strategy with *"the overarching goals of increasing life expectancy and reducing inequalities"* (*Position Paper*, 2003 p 9).

School nurses will be commissioned within the GMS (General Medical Services) Contract such that they can demonstrate collaboration between trusts and within primary care. The Community Nursing Strategy is a sub strategy of the Strategy for Primary Care.

Referring to England's *Liberating the Talents* (2003), first contact care; chronic disease management/continuing care; and public health are re-sited in the NI strategy such that (1) population need (e.g., children) and (2) how their needs can be met become the fundamental orientation for practice.

Also affecting school nurse practice in Northern Ireland is the commitment to a review of nurse education for nurses working in the community and primary care. *"Job descriptions will become more important in defining what community nurses do."* (*Position Paper*, 2003, p 13). To support this, post registration education and development for community nurses is being developed across the four countries of the UK in a consistent fashion in order to allow freedom of movement of nurses pursuing their careers across the UK (the Nursing and Midwifery Council Code of Conduct). The Northern Ireland strategy is explicitly committed to an incremental build up of skills and school nurse practice will be contained within the community nursing strategy.

The message for school nurse practice in Northern Ireland is consistent with the trajectory of change we have found elsewhere: a social model of care that is firmly rooted in public health practice and a practice model that is based on skill-mix and cross-departmental working.

4 RECOMMENDATIONS FOR 'NEXT STEPS' RESEARCH

`School nurse practice needs impact and outcome measures in order to argue for appropriate funding levels and for service development. In order to establish such measures, services need to specify their activities and their target outcomes for child health improvement.

School nurse services need to consult children, young people and their families about their health needs and the kinds of services they wish to receive and will use. The methods and outcomes of such consultations need to be published for transfer across services.

There is need for large-scale and comparative studies of school nurse practice development across and within the four countries of the UK.

School nurse leadership has never been studied despite its critical importance in the development of practice over the past decade. There is need for research into this aspect of service delivery.

References

> *Additional literature: please send to*
> ddebell@compuserve.com

Adams A., Amos L., Munro J. (eds) (2002) *Promoting Health: Politics and Practice*. Sage Publications: London.

Adelman H., Taylor L., Bradley B., Lewis K. (1997) Mental health in schools. Expanded opportunities for school nurses. *Journal of School Nursing* 13, 6-12.

ADDS Children and Families Committee (2002) *Tomorrow's children*. Association of Directors of Social Services: London.

Aggleton P. and Campbell C. (2000) Working with young people – towards an agenda for sexual health. *Sexual and Relationship Therapy* 15:3, 283-296.

Allensworth D.D. (1996) Guidelines for Adolescent Preventive Services: a role for the school nurse. *Journal of School Health* 66:8, 281-285.

Anderton J., Broady J. (October 27,1999) Improving schools' asthma policies and procedures. *Nursing Standard* 14:6, 34-38.

Audit Commission (1994) *Seen but not heard: co-ordinating community child health and social services for children in need*. HMSO: Norwich.

Audit Commission (1999) *children in mind: child and adolescent mental health services*. The Audit Commission: London. www.audit-commission.gov.uk

Aynsley-Green A., Barker M., Burr S., Macfarlane A., Morgan J., Silbert J., Turner T., Viner R., Watson T., Hall D. (2000) Who is speaking for children and adolescents and for their health at policy level? *British Medical Journal* 321, 229-232.

Bagnall P. (1997) The dangers of cutting school nursing services. *Nursing Times* 93:24, 58-59.

Bagnall P. and Dilloway M. (1996) *In A Different Light. School Nurses and Their Role in Meeting the Needs of School Age Children*. Department of Health: London.

Bagnall P. and Dilloway M. (1996) *In search of a blueprint: a survey of school health services*. The Queen's Nursing Institute: London.

Balding J (2001) *Young People in 2000: The Health-related Behaviour Questionnaire Results for 42,073 Young People Between the Ages of 10 and 15*. School Health Education Unit: Exeter.

Ball J. and Pike G. (July 2005) *School Nurses: Results from a census survey of RCN school nurses in 2005*. Employment Research Ltd and RCN: London.

Baraitser P., Dolan F., Cowley S. (2003) Developing relationships between sexual health clinics and schools: more than clinic nurses doing sex education sessions? *Sex Education* 3:3, 201-213.

Baraitser P. and Wood A. (2001) Precarious partnerships: barriers to multidisciplinary sex education in schools. *Health Education Journal* 60, 127-131.

Baptiste L. and Drennan V. (December/January 1999) Communication between school nurses and primary care teams. *British Journal of Community Nursing* 4:1, 13-18.

Barlow J., Stewart Brown S., Fletcher J. (1997) *Systematic review of the school entry medical examination*. Health Services Research Unit, University of Oxford: Oxford.

Bates A. and Wheatley M. (April 1998) School nursing: Managing a BCG administration programme. *Community Practitioner* 71:4, 136-137.

Bax M. and Whitmore K. (1991) Every child should have one. *Health visitor* 64:5, 157-159.

Bedford H., Elliman D., and Hugman J. (January 2004) Screening in childhood. *Community Practitioner* 77:1, 7-9. (See Elliman, Bedford, Hugman below.)

Bekaer S. (November 2002) School nurses and sexual health education. *JCN Online* 16:11, 9 pages. www.jcn.co.uk/journal.asp?MonthNum=11&YearNum=2002&ArticleID=529

Bekemeier B. (1995) Public health nurses and the prevention of and intervention in family violence. *Public Health Nursing* 12, 222 -227.

Billings J. (1998) A long time coming. *Nursing Times* 94:28, 30-31.

Billingham K. (1997) Public health nursing in primary care. *British Journal of Community Health Nursing* 2:6, 270-274.

Blair M., Stewart Brown S., Waterson T., Crowther R. (2003) *Children's Public Health*. Oxford University Press: Oxford.

Boon A., Lynch M., Macfarlane A., Waterston T. (1997) The Essentials of Community Health Services for Children and Young People. *Report of a Working Party*. RCPCH: London.

Borup I.K. (1998) Pupils' experiences of the annual health dialogue with the school health nurse. *Scandinavian Journal of Caring Sciences* 12:3, 160-169.

Bowen C. (March 2000) Taking school nursing into the community. *Nursing Times* 96:11, 43.

Bradley B.J. (February 1998) Establishing a research agenda for school nursing. *Journal of School Health* 68:2, 53-61.

British Medical Association Board of Science and Education (2003) *Adolescent Health*. BMA: London.

British Paediatric Association (November 1991) *Towards a Combined Child Health Service*. BPA: London.

Brown T. (1996) *Opportunities for health and education to work together: Lining the Health of the Nation targets to the National Curriculum*. NHS Executive: South Thames Regional Health Authority.

Bolton A. (1997) *Losing the Thread: Pupils' and Parents' Voices About Education for Sick Children*. National Association for the Education of Sick Children: London.

Bowen C. (1996) Educating teachers in children's illnesses: a study. *Nursing Standard* 10, 33-39.

Broomfield D.M. and Tew J. (1992) Selective medicals at school entry. *Public Health* 106:2, 149-154.

Buchan J. (2000) *Summary Nursing Labour Markets in Europe: Planning for Change*. World Health Organization Regional Office for Europe: Geneva.

Buckland L., Rose J., Greaves C. (January 2005) New roles for school nurses: preventing exclusion. *Community practitioner* 78:1, 16-19.

Buttigieg M. (2003) *Redesign of Services to School Age Children in Lewisham*. MAB Consulting. Lewisham PCT: London.

Buttigieg M. (2001) *Looking Ahead: Towards A Strategy for School Nursing*. North Hampshire Hospitals NHS Trust Children's Services: North Hampshire.

Buttigieg M. (2001) *School Nurses Are Not Just for Schools: A review of school nursing services in Lambeth*. Community Health South London NHS Trust: London.

Caulfield H. (September 1997) Legal aspects of consent for school nurses. *Primary Health Care* 7:7, 28-29.

Center for Children with Special Needs (June 2001) *School Nurse Outcome Measures*. Washington State Office of Superintendent of Public Instruction: Washington State USA.

Chapman S.K. and Stewart Brown S. (1998) *The school entry check: the literature*. Health Services Research Unit, University of Oxford: Oxford.

Charleston S. and Denman S. (August 1997) The school nurse's contribution to health promotion. *Health visitor* 70:8, 302-304.

Charlesworth J. (2001) Negotiating and managing partnership in primary care. *Health and Social Care in the Community* 9:5, 279-289.

Chattaway S. *Developing and implementing a strategy for East Cheshire School Health Service using a whole systems approach*. East Cheshire School Health Service: Macclesfield.

Children & Young People's Unit (2001) *Building a strategy for children & young people*. CYPU: London.

Children's Society, National Children's Bureau, Barnardo's and NCH (2001) *Improving Children's Health (2) – An Analysis of Health Improvement Programmes (2000-2003)*. NSPCC: London.

Clark A. (June 2004) The role of the school nurse in tackling childhood obesity. *Nursing Times* 100:23.

Clark D.J., Buttigieg M., Bodycombe-James M., Eaton N., Kelly A., Merrell J., Palmer-Thomas J., Parke S., Symonds A. (April 2000) *Recognising the Potential: A Review of Health Visiting and School Health Services in Wales*. School of Health Science, University of Wales: Cardiff.

Clarke M. Out of the Wilderness and Into the Fold: The School Nurse and Child Protection. *Child Abuse Review* 9, 364-374.

Clarke M., Coombs C., Walton L. (2003) School based early identification and intervention service for adolescents: A Psychology and School Nurse Partnership Model. *Child and Adolescent Mental Health* 8:1, 34-39.

Cleaver H., Barnes J., Bliss D., Cleaver D. (2004) *Developing identification, referral and tracking systems: an evaluation of the processes undertaken by trailblazer authorities – early findings*. DfES: London.

Cleaver H., Walker S., Meadows P. (2004) *Assessing children's needs and circumstances: the impact of the assessment framework*. Jessica Kingsley Publishers: London.

Coles P. (April 1998) Linking with primary health and voluntary sector services. *Healthy Minds* 1, 4-5.

Commission on Nursing (1998) *The Report of the Commission on Nursing: A blueprint for the future*. The Stationery Office: Dublin.

Community Practitioners' and Health Visitors' Association (1997) *Public health: the role of nurses and health visitors*. CPHVA: London.

Community Practitioners' and Health Visitors' Association (2001) *Actions taken by the CPHVA concerning the Review of the Nursing, Midwifery and Health Visiting Act of 1979 and its results*. CPHVA: London.

Community Practitioners' and Health Visitors' Association, Community Psychiatric Nurses' Association and Manufacturing, Science and Finance (September 2001) *Community Values – Valuing the Community: Profiling Community Nursing*. CPHVA: London.

Community Practitioners and Health Visitors' Association (1998) *Healthy futures: the diversity of school nursing*. CPHVA: London.

Community Practitioners and Health Visitors' Association (1998) *The principles of school nursing: Foundations of good practice*. CPHVA: London.

Community Practitioners and Health Visitors' Association (1999) *Joined Up Working. Community Development in Primary Healthcare*. CPHVA: London.

Connelly J. and Worth C. (1997) *Making Sense of Public Health Medicine*. Radcliffe Medical Press: Oxford.

Cooke J., Owen J., Wilson A. (2002) Research and development at the health and social care interface in primary care: a scoping exercise in one NHS region. *Social Policy and Administration* 10:6, 435-444.

Coote A., Allen J., Woodhead D. (November 2004) *Finding Out What Works: Understanding complex, community-based initiatives*. King's Fund: London.

Costello J. and Haggart M. (eds) (2003) *Public Health and Society*. Palgrave Macmillan: Basingstoke.

Cotton L., Brazier J., Hall D.M.B., Lindsay G., Marsh P., Polnay L., Williams T.S. (May 2000) School nursing: costs and potential benefits. *Journal of Advanced Nursing* 31:5, 1063-1071.

Court D. (1976) *Fit for the Future*. UK Commission of Enquiry into the Child Health Services: London.

Cowley S. (1999) From population to people: public health in practice. *Community practitioner* 72:4, 88-90.

Cowley S. (ed) (2002) *Public Health in Policy and Practice*. Balliere Tindall: London.

Cowley S. (ed) (forthcoming 2006) *Community public health, policy and practice: a source book*. Elsevier: London.

Cowley S., Houston A.M. (2003) A structured health needs assessment tool: acceptability and effectiveness for health visiting. *Journal of Advanced Nursing* 43, 1847-1851.

Cowley S., Buttigieg M. and Houston A. (April 2000) *A First Steps Approach to Scope the Current and Future Regulatory Issues for Health Visiting: Report for the United Kingdom Central Council for Nursing, Midwifery and Health Visiting*. King's College London: London.

Crown J. (200) *Nursing and Midwifery for Health21*. World Health Organization Regional office for Europe: Copenhagen,

Coverdale G. (February 2005) School nurses in the spotlight. *Community practitioner* 78:2, 48-49.

Craig P.M. and Lindsey G.M. (eds) (2000) *Nursing for Public Health: Population Based Care*. Churchill Livingstone: London.

Croghan E. (2002) A survey of drinking and toilet facilities in local state schools. *British Journal of Community Nursing* 7:2, 76-79.

Croghan E. and Johnson C. (January 2004) Occupational health and school health: a natural alliance? *Journal of Advanced Nursing* 45:2, 155-161.

Croghan E., Johnson C., Aveyard P. (2004) School nurses: policies, working practices, roles and value perceptions. *Journal of Advanced Nursing* 47:4, 377-385.

Crouch V. (1999) Sex and the school nurse. *Nursing Standard* 13:36, 16-17.

Crouch V. (2002) Teenage pregnancy, better prevention and a sexual health game for young people. *Education and Health* 20:1, 13-16.

Cullum K.L. (May 2005) *School Based Sex Education — The Role of the School Nurse: A Review and Critical Analysis of Relevant Literature*. BSc dissertation (unpublished). University of East Anglia: Norwich.

Currie C., Roberts C., Morgan A., Smith R., Settertobulte W., Samdal O., Rasmussen V.B. (eds) (2004) Young people's health in context. Health Behaviour in School-aged Children (HBSC) Study: International report from the 2001/2002 survey. *Health Policy for Children and Adolescents, No. 4*. World Health Organization Regional Office for Europe: Copenhagen. www.euro.who.int/InformationSources/Publications/Catalogue/20040601_1?Print

Currie J. and Lyttle P. (December 2004) Teenage sexual health promotion: the Dumfries and Galloway perspective. *Community practitioner* 77:12, 450-452.

Davis B. and McIntyre F. (1997) Pilot of a questionnaire for parents of school entrants. *Health visitor* 69:10, 298-299.

Davis C., Finlay L., Bullman A. (eds) (2000) *Changing Practice in Health and Social Care*. Sage Publications: London.

Day P. (August 3, 2000) School nurses and contraception. *Nursing Times* 96:31, 39-40.

DeBell D. and Everett G. (1996) The role and function of the school nurse. *British Journal of Community Health Nursing* 1:8, 486-493.

DeBell D. and Everett G. (1997) *In A Class Apart: A Study of School Nursing*. City College: Norwich.

DeBell D. and Everett G. (May 1998) The changing role of school nursing within health education and health promotion. *Health Education* 98:3, 107-115.

DeBell D. and Jackson P. (2000) *School nursing within the public health agenda – a strategy for practice*. Community Practitioners and Health Visitors Association, Queens Nursing Institute, Royal College of Nursing. McMillan-Scott: London.

DeBell D. (February 1998) Guest Editorial: The challenge of leadership in community nursing. *British Journal of Community Nursing* 3:2, 62-63.

DeBell D. (6 June 2000) Singing the praises of the school nurse. *Guardian Education Supplement, 7*.

DeBell D. (2000) *The Health Promoting Role of School Nursing. A Review: North Staffordshire*. Centre for Research in Health and Social Care, Anglia Ruskin University: Chelmsford and Cambridge.

DeBell D (2003) *North Bradford PCT: School Nursing Review*. Centre for Research in Health and Social Care, Anglia Ruskin University: Chelmsford and Cambridge.

Denehy J. (June 2003) Developing a Program of Research in School Nursing: Editorial. *The Journal of School Nursing* 19:3, 125-126.

Denman S. (1994) Do schools provide an opportunity for meeting the Health of the Nation targets? *Journal of Public Health Medicine* 16:2, 219-224.

Denman S., Reeves J., Arnold R., Pearce R. (1995) *Sex, contraception and parenthood. A study of young women's knowledge and attitudes in Nottingham*. A report to Nottingham. Department of Public Health Medicine and Epidemiology, University of Nottingham: Nottingham.

Department for Education and Employment and Department of Health (1997) *Supporting Pupils with Medical Needs: A good practice guide*. DfEE and Department of Health: London.

Department for Education and Employment (1999) *The National Healthy School Standard Guidance*. DfEE: London. www.Standards.dfes.gov.uk/sie/si/SgCC/goodpractice/nhss

Department for Education and Employment (2000) *Sex and Relationships Guidance*. DfEE: London.

Department for Education and Employment (2001) *Access to Education for Children and Young People with Medical Needs.* DfES 0732/2001, DfES Publications: Nottingham. www.dfes.gov.uk/Sickchildren/Pdfs/Accesstoed.pdf

Department for Education and Environment (1997) *Excellence in schools.* DfEE: London.

Department for Education and Environment (1999) *National Healthy Schools Standard – Getting Started.* DfEE: London. www.Standards.dfes.gov.uk/sie/si/SgCC/goodpractice/nhss

Department for Education and Skills (2001a) *Connexions for all – working to provide a service for all young people.* DfES: Nottingham. www.connexions.gov.uk/partnerships/publications

Department for Education and Skills (2001b) *Promoting children's mental health within early years and schools settings.* DfES: London. www.teachernet.gov.uk/_doc/3718/UPDATE%208.htm

Department for Education and Skills, Department of Health and Home Office (2003) *Keeping Children Safe: The Government's Response to the Victoria Climbie Inquiry Report and Joint Chief Inspectors' Report Safeguarding Children.* HMSO: Norwich. www.everychildmatters.gov.uk/publications/?asset=document&ID=19540

Department for Education and Skills (2004b) *Every child matters: change for children.* DfES: London. www.dfes.gov.uk/everychildmatters/

Department for Education and Skills (2004c) *Every child matters: next steps.* Department for Education and Skills Publications: Nottingham. www.everychildmatters.gov.uk/_files/A39928055378AF27E9122D734BF10F74.pdf and www.everychildmatters.gov.uk/strategy/planningandcommissioning/cypp/

Department for Education and Skills (2004d) *Every Child Matters: Change for Children in Schools.* DfES: London. www.everychildmatters.gov.uk/publications/?asset=document&ID=15549

Department for Education and Skills and the Department of Health (2004e) *National Healthy Schools Programme.* DfES: London. www.wiredforhealth.gov.uk

Department of Education and Skills (2005) *Managing Medicines in Schools and Early Years Settings.* DfES: Nottingham.

Department for Education and Skills (July 2005) *Youth Matters.* HMSO: Norwich. www.dfes.gov.uk/publications/youth/

Department for Education and Skills (October 2005) *Higher Standards, Better Schools for All – More choice for Parents and Pupils.* HMSO: Norwich. www.dfes.gov.uk/publications

Department of Health and Children Dublin (2000) *The National Health Promotion Strategy 2000 - 2005.* DOHC: Dublin. www.dohc.ie/publications/national_health_promotion_strategy.html

Department of Health and Social Security (1986) *Neighbourhood Nursing: A Focus for Care. Cumberlege Report.* HMSO: Norwich.

Department of Health (1992) *The Health of the Nation Strategy for Health in England and Wales.* CM1986. HMSO: Norwich.

Department of Health (1993) *Children Act Report 1993 — Children Act 1989: A Report to the Secretaries of State for Health and for Wales on the Children Act 1989 in pursuance of their duties under Section 83(6) of the Act.* HMSO: London.

Department of Health (1994) *Negotiating school health services.* HMSO: London.

Department of Health (1995) *Child Protection: Messages from Research.* Studies in Child Protection. HMSO: London.

Department of Health (1995b) *Nurses and purchasing. Change, challenge, opportunity: school nurses in the new health service structure.* HMSO: London.

Department of Health (1996a) *Child Health in the Community: a Guide to Good Practice.* NHS Executive: London. www.dh.gov.uk/assetRoot/04/01/24/50/04012450.pdf

Department of Health (1996b) *The Patient's Charter – services for children and young people.* HMSO: Norwich.

Department of Health (1997a) *Making It Happen: Public Health – The Contribution, Role and Development of Nurses, Midwives and Health Visitors.* Leaflet based on 1995 report. Report of the Standing Nursing and Midwifery Advisory Committee and the NHS Executive. Department of Health: London. www.dh.gov.uk/AdvancedSearch/SearchResults/fs/en?PG=1&RP=20&NP=5& . . .

Department of Health (1997b) *The New NHS: Modern and Dependable.* HMSO: Norwich. www.officialdocuments.co.uk/document/doh/newnhs/newnhs.htm

Department of Health (1998a) *The New NHS Modern and Dependable: a national framework for assessing performance.* NHS Executive: London. www.dh.gov.uk/assetRoot/04/01/13/87/04011387.pdf

Department of Health (1998b) *Our Healthier Nation: A Contract for Health. Consultation Green Paper.* HMSO: Norwich. www.official-documents.co.uk/document/doh/ohnation/title.htm

Department of Health (1998c) *Report of the Independent Inquiry into Inequalities in Health.* HMSO: Norwich. www.official-documents.co.uk/document/doh/ih/contents.htm

Department of Health (1998d) *Working together: securing a quality workforce for the NHS.* Department of Health: London. www.dh.gov.uk/assetRoot/04/01/44/84/040/4484.pdf

Department of Health (1999a) *The Government's Response to the Health Committee's Report on Future Staffing Requirements.* Department of Health: London.

Department of Health (1999b) *Making a difference: Strengthening the nursing, midwifery and health visiting contribution to health and healthcare.* HMSO: Norwich. www.dh.gov.uk/PublicationsAndStatistics/Publications/PublicationsPolicyAndGuidance/PublicationsPolicyAndGuidanceArticle/

Department of Health (1999c) *Opportunities in nursing, midwifery and health visiting: Building a career in health care.* Department of Health: London.

Department of Health (1999d) *Partnership in Action: Opportunities for Joint Working between Health and Social Services.* HMSO: Norwich. www.dh.gov.uk/assetRoot/04/ 01/44/88/04014488.pdf

Department of Health (1999e) *Saving Lives: Our Healthier Nation.* HMSO: Norwich. www.doh.gov.uk/ohn.htm

Department of Health (1999f) *Working together to safeguard children.* HMSO: Norwich. www.dh.gov.uk/assetRoot/04/07/ 58/24/04075824.pdf

Department of Health (2000a) *Human Resources Performance Framework.* Department of Health: London. www.dh.gov.uk/assetRoot/04/01/22/62/04-12262.pdf

Department of Health (2000b) *Modernising Regulation: The New Nursing and Midwifery Council: A Consultation Document.* Department of Health: London.

Department of Health (2000c) *The NHS Plan: A Plan for Investment. A Plan for Reform.* HMSO: Norwich. www.doh.gov.uk/nhsplan/nhsplan.htm

Department of Health (2000d) *Tackling Teenage Pregnancy: Action for Health Authorities and Local Authorities.* Teenage Pregnancy Unit: London.

Department of Health (2000e) *Towards a Strategy for Nursing Research and Development.* Department of Health: London. www.dh.gov.uk/assetRoot/04/07/66/47/04076647.pdf

Department of Health (2001a) *Establishing the Nursing and Midwifery Council.* Department of Health: London.

Department of Health (2001b) *From Vision to Reality.* Department of Health: London. www.dh.gov.uk/assetRoot/04/05/94/59/04059459.pdf

Department of Health (2001c) *Government Response to the House of Commons Select Committee on Health's Second Report on Public Health.* Department of Health: London. www.dh.gov.uk/assetRoot/04/08/21/36/04082136.pdf

Department of Health (2001d) *The Health Visitor and School Nurse Development Programme: School nurse practice development resource pack.* HMSO: Norwich. www.dh.gov.uk/assetRoot/04/05/08/37/04050837.pdf

Department of Health (2001e) *Making a Difference in Primary Care: The challenge for nurses, midwives and health visitors. Case Studies from NHS Regional Conferences.* Department of Health: London. www.dh.gov.uk/assetRoot/04/05/08/37/ 04050837.pdf

Department of Health (2001f) *Making it happen: a guide to delivering mental health promotion.* HMSO: Norwich. www.dh.gov.uk/assetRoot/04/05/89/58/04058958.pdf

Department of Health (2001g) *School Nurse Practice Development Resource Pack.* Department of Health: London.

Department of Health (2001h) *Shifting the Balance of Power within the NHS: securing delivery.* HMSO: Norwich. www.doh.gov.uk/publications/pointh.html

Department of Health (2001i) *Smoking, Drinking and Drug Use among Young People in England 2000.* HMSO: Norwich. www.dh.gov.uk/PublicationsAndStatistics/PressReleases/ PressReleasesNotices/fs/en%3

Department of Health (2001j) *Working Together Under the Act.* HMSO: Norwich.

Department of Health (2002a) *National Healthy School Standard School Nursing.* Health Development Agency: Wetherby.

Department of Health (2002b) *National Suicide Prevention Strategy for England.* HMSO: Norwich. www.dh.gov.uk/ assetRoot/ 04/01/95/48/04019548.pdf

Department of Health (2002c) *Safeguarding Children. A Joint Chief Inspectors' report on arrangements to safeguard children.* Department of Health: London. www.dh.gov.uk/assetRoot/04/01/12/92/04011292.pdf

Department of Health (September 2003a) *Every Child Matters.* HMSO: Norwich. www.everychildmatters.gov.uk

Department of Health (2003b) *Liberating the Talents. Helping Primary Care Trusts and Nurses to Deliver the NHS Plan.* HMSO: Norwich. www.dh.gov.uk/assetRoot/04/07/62/50/ 04076250.pdf

Department of Health (2003c)*Tackling Health Inequalities – A Programme for Action.* Department of Health: London. www.doh.gov.uk/healthinequalities/programmeforaction

Department of Health (2004c) *The Chief Nursing Officer's review of the nursing, midwifery and health visiting contribution to vulnerable children and young people.* Department of Health: London. www.gov.dh.gov.uk/ assetRoot/04/08/72/21/04087221.pdf

Department of Health and Department for Education and Skills (2004) *National Service Framework for Children, Young People and Maternity Services.* HMSO: Norwich. www.dh.gov.uk/assetRoot/04/09/05/52/04090552. pdf and www.dh.gov.uk/PolicyAndGuidance/ HealthAndSocialCareTopics/ChildrenServices/Children ServicesInformation/ChildrenServicesInformationArticle/fs/ en?CONTENT_ID=4089111&chk=U8Ecln

Department of Health (2005) *Delivering choosing health.* Department of Health: London. www.dh.gov.uk/PublicationsAndStatistics/PublicationsPolicy AndGuidance/PublicationsPolicyAndGuidanceArticle/ fs/en?CONTENT_ID=4105355&chk=gFTjxL

DiCenso A., Guyatt G., Willan A., Griffith L. (15 June 2002) Interventions to reduce unintended pregnancies among adolescents: systematic review of randomised controlled trials. *British Medical Journal* 324, 1426-1430.

Dombrowski A.M. (March 1999) Preventing disease with stress management in elementary schools. *Journal of School Health* 69:3, 126-127.

Donovan C., Parry-Langdon N., Richardson G., Jacobson L. (2001a) *Bridging the Gap: A Descriptive Study of Communication with Teenagers in General Practice.* University of Wales College of Cardiff: Cardiff.

Donovan C., Parry-Langdon N., Richardson G., Jacobson L. (2001b) Teenagers' views on the general practice consultation and provision of contraception. *British Journal of General Practice* 47, 715-718.

Downie R.S., Tannahill C. and Tannahill A. (1996 2nd edition) *Health Promotion: Models and Values*. Oxford Medical Publications: Oxford.

Duffin C. (December 2000) Calling all the shots: The rules about consent to treatment are not always clear, especially for nurses working with children. *Nursing Standard* 15:1, 12-13.

Dunnett K., Barnet T., Belcher A., Gibson D., Ives T., Nicholls A., Souther I., Walton J. (January 2005) *Partnership Working: If it is so easy, why aren't we all doing it?* Community Practitioners' and Health Visitors' Association: London.

Dyson A., Lin M., Millward A. (1998) *Communication Between Schools, LEAs and Health and Social Services in the Field of Special Educational Needs*. Special Needs Research Centre, University of Newcastle: Newcastel upon Tyne.

Edwards L.H. (June 2002) Research Priorities in School Nursing: A Delphi Process. *The Journal of School Nursing* 18:3, 157-162.

El Ansai W., Phillips C.J., Hammick M. (2001) Collaboration and Partnerships: Developing the Evidence Base. *Health and Social Care in the Community* 9:4, 215-233.

Ellefsen B. (1998a) Cooperation in community health nursing. *Nursing Leadership Forum* 3:2, 74-80.

Ellefsen B. (1998b) Influence and leadership in community-based nursing in Norway. *Public Health Nursing* 15:5, 348-354.

Ellefsen B. (August 2002) School nursing in Scotland and Norway compared. *Community practitioner* 75:8, 299-303.

Elliman D., Bedford H., Hugman J. (February 2004) Newborn and childhood screening programmes: part two. *Community practitioner* 77:2, 41-43. (See Bedford, Elliman, Hugman above.)

Elliott L., Crombie I.K., Irvine L., Cantrell J., Taylor J. (2001) *Nursing for Health: The Effectiveness of Public Health Nursing: A Review of Systematic Reviews*. Scottish Executive and University of Dundee: Dundee.

Elston S. and Holloway I. (2001) The impact of recent primary care reforms in the UK on interprofessional working in primary care centres. *Journal of Interprofessional Care* 15:1, 19-27.

Exworthy M., Stuart M., Blane D., Marmot M. (March 2003) *Tackling health inequalities since the Acheson Inquiry*. Joseph Rowntree Foundation. The Policy Press: Bristol.

Evans D. (September 2000) From 'nits' to 'crabs'?: school nurses and sexual health. *British Journal of Nursing* 9:18, 2022-2023.

Evans D. (2003) 'Taking public health out of the ghetto': the policy and practice of multidisciplinary public health in the United Kingdom. *Social Science and Medicine* 57, 959-967.

Farrell J. (1998) Asthma and school nursing: An asthma management project in Wakefield schools. *Professional Care of Mother & Child* 8:1, 12-14.

Farrow S. (2001) The Role of the School Nurse in Promoting Health. In Scriven A. and Crome J. (eds 2nd ed) *Health Promotion. Professional Perspectives*. Palgrave in association with The Open University: Hampshire.

Few C.M., Hicken I., Butterworth A.C. (1995) *Developing healthy alliances between school nurses and teachers in HIV, STD and sex education in secondary schools*. School of nursing studies, University of Manchester: Manchester.

Fletcher J., Brown S., Barlow J. (1997) *Systematic review of reviews of the effectiveness of school health promotion*. Health Services Research Unit, Oxford University: Oxford.

Fonagy P., Target M., Cottrell D., Phillips J., Kurtz Z. (2002) *What Works for Whom? A Critical Review of Treatments for Children and Adolescents*. Guilford: New York.

Gleeson C. (November 2001) Children's access to school health nurses. *Primary Health Care* 11:9, 33-36.

Gleeson C. (2001) A review of teenagers' perceived needs and access to primary health care. *Primary Health Care* 11:9, 33-36.

Gleeson C. (2003) Improving teenagers' access to health services. *Practice Nursing* 14:6, 263-266.

Gleeson C. (April 2004) School health nursing – evidence-based practice? *Primary Health Care* 14:3, 38-41.

Gleeson C., Robinson M., Neal R. (2002) A review of teenagers' perceived needs and access to primary health care: Implications for health services. *Primary Health Care Research and Development* 3, 184-193.

Glisson C. and Hemmelgarn A. (1998) The effects of organizational climate and interorganizational coordination on the quality and outcomes of children's service systems. *Child Abuse and Neglect* 22:5, 401-421.

Grant A.H. (1942) *Nursing: a community health service*. W.B. Saunders Co.: Philadelphia.

Greenhaulgh S. (1997) Improving schoolteachers' knowledge of diabetes. *Professional Nurse* 13, 150-156.

Griffiths S. and Hunter D. (1999) *Perspectives in public health*. Radcliffe Medical Press: Oxford.

Grimsmo A. (1989) *Health prevention for school-age children*. Kommuneforlagett: Oslo.

Guillebaud J. (1998) Time for emergency contraception with levonorgestrel alone. *The Lancet* 352:9126, 416-417.

Hacker K. and Wessel G.L. (1998) School-based health centres and school nurses: cementing the collaboration. *Journal of School Health* 68:10, 98-100.

Hadley A. (1999) Improving teenage sexual health: how nurses can help. *Primary Health Care* 9:1, 6-11.

Hall C. and Milner P. (1996) Advertising emergency contraception using local radio. An evaluation. *Health Education Journal* 55, 165-174.

Hall D. (ed) (1996) *Health for all children. Report of the Third Joint Working Party on Child Health Surveillance*. Third edition. Oxford University Press: Oxford.

Hall D.M.B. (August 1999) School nursing: Past, present and future. *Archives of Disease in Childhood* 81:2, 181-184.

Hall D.M.B. and Elliman D. (ed.) (2003, 4th edition, updated reprint forthcoming June 2006) *Health for all children*. Oxford University Press: Oxford. www.health-for-all-children.co.uk .

Hamilton K. and Saunders L. (1997) *The health promoting school: a summary of the ENHPS evaluation project in England*. National Foundation for Educational Research. Health Education Authority: London.

Harris B. (1995) *The health of the schoolchild*. Open University Press: Buckingham.

Harrison A., Gretton J. (1986) School health: the invisible service. In Harrison A., Gretton J. (eds) *Health care UK 1986*. Policy Journals. Hermitage: Berkshire.

Harrison S. (17 August 2005) I want to hear from you: Nurses are invited to tell England's new commissioner for children what his main priorities should be. *Nursing Standard* 19:49, 14-15.

Health Advisory Service (1995) *Together we stand: Child and adolescent mental health services*. HMSO: London.

Health Development Agency (July 2004) *The Health Visitor and School Nurse Innovations Network*. innovate.had-online.org.uk/default.asp

Health Visitors' Association (1995) *Action for School Health: an HVA guide*. HVA: London.

Health Visitors' Association (1996) *School nursing: here today for tomorrow*. HVA: London.

Henderson S (1999) *Supporting Parenting in Scotland*. Social Work Research Findings No 33: Scottish Office. *Journal of School Health* 67, 327-332.

Heneghan A. and Malakoff M. (1997) Availability of school health services for young children. *Journal of School Health* 67, 327-332.

Henshelwood J. and Polnay L., (1994) Facilities for the school health team. *Archives of Disease in Childhood* 70, 542-544.

Higher Education Funding Council for England (2001) *Research in nursing and the allied health professions: Report of the Task Group 3 to HEFCE and the Department of Health*. HEFCE: Bristol. www.hefce.ac.uk/Pubs/hefce/2001/0163.htm

Hiscock J. and Pearson M. (1999) Looking inward, looking outward. Dismantling the 'Berlin Wall' between health and social services. *Social Policy and Administration* 33:2, 150-163.

Holland W.W. (1998) *Public Health. The Vision and the Challenge*. The Nuffield Trust: London.

Home Office (1998) *Supporting families*. HMSO: Norwich.

Home Office (2003) *Hidden Harm – Responding to the needs of children of problem drug users, the report of an inquiry by the Advisory Council on the Misuse of Drugs*. Home Office: London. www.homeoffice.gov.uk/docs2/hiddenharm.html

House of Commons (1997) *Health Services for Children and Young People in the Community: home and school*. Third Report from the Health Committee HC 314-I. HMSO: Norwich.

Houghton A., Egan S., Archinal G., Bradley O., Azam N. (1992) Selective medical examination at school entry: should we do it, and if so how? *Journal of Public Health Medicine* 14:2, 111-116.

Humphries J. and Tonge J. (2000) Looking ahead: a forum on the future of school nursing. *Community practitioner* 73:12, 881-883.

Humphries J. (9 January 2002) The school nurse and health education in the classroom. *Nursing Standard* 16:17, 42-45.

Hudson B. (1999) Dismantling the 'Berlin Wall' development at the health and social care interface. *Social Policy Review* 11, 187-204.

Hudson B. (2000) Social services and Primary Care Groups: a window of collaborative opportunity? *Health and Social Care in the Community* 8:4, 242-250.

Hudson B. (2002) Interprofessionality in health and social care:the Achilles' heel of partnership? *Journal of Interprofessional Care* 16:3, 199-210.

Hudson F. and West J. (1996) Needing to be heard. The young person's agenda. *Education and Health* 14:3, 43-47.

Igoe J. (1994) School Nursing. *Nursing Clinics of North America* 29, 443-458.

Ingham R. (1999) *Teenage sexual knowledge, attitudes and behaviour in England*. Department of Psychology: University of Southampton.

Jackson C. (1996) Here today for tomorrow. *Health visitor* 69:10, 403-404.

Jacobson L., Richardson G., Parry-Langdon N., Donovan C. (2001) How do teenagers and primary healthcare providers view each other? An overview of key themes. *British Journal of General Practice* 51, 811-816.

Jamison J., Ashby P., Hamilton K., Lewis G., Macdonald A., Saunders L. (1998) *The health promoting school. Final report of the ENHPS evaluation project in England*. Health Education Authority: London.

Jewell C. (2004) *Can the School Nurse Identify and Alleviate Stress in Primary School Children?* Internal Paper submitted for the BMedSci in Specialist School Nursing. Sheffield University: Sheffield.

J.M. Consulting Ltd (1998) *The Regulation of Nurses, Midwives and Health Visitors: Report on a review of the Nurses, Midwives and Health Visitors Act 1997*. J.M. Consulting: Bristol.

Johnson M., Mercer C.H., Erens B., Copas A.J., McManus S., Wellings K., Fenton K.A., Korovessis C., Macdowall W., Nanchahal K., Purdon S., Field J. (1 December 2001) Sexual behaviour in Britain: partnerships, practices, and HIV risk behaviours. *The Lancet* 358, 1835-1842.

Johnson P., Wistow G., Scullz R., Hardy B. (2003) Interagency and interprofessional collaboration in community care: the interdependence of structures and values. *Journal of Interprofessional Care* 17:1, 69-83.

Jones D. (2001) The Assessment of Parental Capacity. In Howarth J. (ed.) *The child's world: assessing children in need.* Jessica Kingsley Publishers: London.

Jones R., Finlay F., Simpson N., Kreitman T. (October 1997) How can adolescents' health needs and concerns best be met? *British Journal of General Practice* 47, 631-634

Jordan J., Wright J., Wilkinson J., Williams R. (1996) *Health Needs Assessment in Primary Care: A Study of the Understanding and Experience in Three Districts.* Nuffield Institute of Health: University of Leeds.

Jowitt S. (2003) *Policy and Practice in Child Welfare: Literature Review Series 3. Child Protection and the Decision-Making Process: Assessments of Risk and Systems of Professional Knowledge, Judgement and Beliefs.* NCH: The Bridge Child Care Development Service. The Bridge Publishing House Ltd.: Glasbury on Wye.

Kari J., Donovan C. Li J., Taylor B. (1998) School and practice nurses – an under-utilised resource. *British Journal of Community Nursing* 3:8, 405-407.

Kazumi T. (1998) *The school health services and school nursing in England.* Miyagi University of Education: Japan.

Kazumi T. (1998) *Trends in school nursing in England.* Miyagi University of Education: Japan.

Kelly A. and Symonds A. (eds) (2003) *The Social Constructs of Community Nursing.* Palgrave Macmillan: Basingstoke.

Kelly N., Greaves C., Buckland L., Rose J. (March 2005) School nurses: well placed to address challenging behaviour. *Community practitioner* 78:3, 88-92.

Kember S., Greengrass J., Walmsley F. (November 1997) *Development of a Health Needs Assessment Process for School Nursing: Assessing the health needs of children and young people of school age.* Norwich Healthcare Partnership NHS Trust: Norwich.

Kennedy F.D. (1988) Have school entry medicals had their day? *Archives of Disease in Childhood* 63:10, 1261-1263.

Kiddy M. and Thurtle V. (August 2002) From chrysalis to butterfly – the school nurse role. *Community practitioner* 75:8, 295-298.

Laing G.J. and Rosser E.B. (September 1998) 'Health assessment' at school entry: Performance of a system based on school nurse interviews. *Care, Health & Development* 25:6, 421-428.

Laming H. (2003) *The Victoria Climbie Inquiry: Report.* HMSO: Norwich.

Lane D. and Day P. (October 2001) Setting up a sexual health clinic in a school. *Nursing Times* 97:41.

Lau B.W.K. (2002) Does the stress in childhood and adolescence matter? A psychological perspective. *The Journal of the Royal Society for the Promotion of Health* 122:4, 238-244.

Leighton S. (2003a) School Nurses and Mental Health. Part 1. *Mental Health Practice* 7:4, 14-16.

Leighton S. (2003b) School Nurses and Mental Health. Part 2. *Mental Health Practice* 7:4, 17-20.

Lightfoot J. and Bines W. (1997) *Keeping Children Healthy: the Role of School Nursing.* Social Policy Research Unit: University of York.

Lightfoot J.and Bines W. (February 1997) Meeting the needs of the school age child. *Health visitor* 70:2, 58-61.*Child: Care, Health & Development* 25:4, 267-283.

Lightfoot J. and Bines W. (1999) *The role of nursing in meeting the health needs of school age children outside hospital. Final report to the Department of Health.* DH1 1430 and Social Policy Research Unit, University of York: York.

Lightfoot J., Wright S., Sloper P. (1998) *Service support for children with a chronic illness or physical disability attending mainstream schools.* NHS1576 and Social Policy Research Unit, University of York: York.

Lightfoot J., Wright S., Sloper P. (1999) Supporting pupils in mainstream school with an illness or disability: young people's views. *Child: Care, Health & Development* 25, 267-283.

Lightfoot J. and Bines W. (March 2000) Working to keep school children healthy: The complementary roles of school staff and school nurses. *Journal of Public Health Medicine* 22:1, 74-80.

Lister-Sharp D., Chapman S., Stewart-Brown S., Sowden A. (1999) Health promoting schools and health promotion in schools: two systematic reviews. *Health Technology Assessment NHS R&D HTA Programme* 3:22, 219pp. www.ncchta.org/fullmono/mon322.pdf

Local Government Association (2004) *From Vision to Reality. Transforming outcomes for children and families.* LGA: London.

Loxley A. (1997) *Collaboration in Health and Welfare. Working with Difference.* Jessica Kingsley Publications: London.

Lupton D. and Tulloch (1996) 'All red in the face': students' views on school-based HIV/AIDS and sexuality education. *Sociological Review* 44, 252-271.

Macduff C. and West J.M. (2003) *Evaluating Family Health Nursing through Education and Practice.* Scottish Executive Social Research, The Scottish Executive: Edinburgh.

Madge H. and Franklin A. *Change, challenge and school nursing.* CPHVA: London.

Mackereth C. (1998) Sexual Health Messages: Working with young people. *Community Practitioner* 71:12, 412-414.

Manthorpe J. and Iliffe S. (2003) Professional predictions: June Huntington's perspectives on joint working, 20 years on. *Journal of Interprofessional Care* 17:1, 85-94.

Maretil R. (June 1998) Goal mouth scramble. *Community Practitioner* 72:6, 172-173.

Mason C. and Clark J (2001) *A Nursing Vision of Public Health: An All Ireland Statement on Public Health and Nursing.* DHSSPS: Belfast and Department of Health and Children: Dublin.

Mayall B., Bendelow G., Barker S., Storey P., Veltman M. (1996) *Children's Health in Primary Schools.* The Falmer Press: London.

Mayall B. and Storey P. (1998) A school health service for children? *Children and Society* 12, 86-97.

Mayer C. (21 June 2001) Sex education for the boys. *Nursing Times* 97:25, 38-39.

Mayes P. and Bays H. (June 1999) Sharing the load: A joint approach to supporting parents. *Community Practioner* 72:6, 172-173.

McDonald A-L., Langford A.H., Boldero N. (1997) The future of community nursing in the United Kingdom: district nursing, health visiting and school nursing. *Journal of Advanced Nursing,* 26, 257-265.

McFadyen J. (2004) Teaching sex education: are Scottish school nurses prepared for the challenge? *Nurse Education Today* 24:2, 113-120.

McKay I. (2003) *The information referral and tracking (IRT) project: issues for implementation in the London Borough of Newham.* Paper 2 PrD (amended). Internal document: Anglia Ruskin University.

McMunn A.M., Nazroo J.Y., Marmot M.G., Boreham R., Goodman R. (2001) Children's emotional and behavioural well-being and the family environment: findings from the Health Survey for England. *Social Science & Medicine* 53, 423-440.

McRae J. and Rote S. (May 1997) Adolescent health: celebrating differences. *Primary Health Care* 7:4, 12-14.

Meltzer H., Gatward R., Goodman R., Ford T. (2000) *Mental health of children and adolescents in Great Britain.* Office for National Statistics. The Stationery Office: London.

Mellanby A.R., Phelps F.A., Crichton N.J., Tripp J.H. (12 August 1995) School Sex Education: an experimental programme with educational and medical benefit. *British Medical Journal* 311, 414-417.

The Mental Health Foundation (1999) *Bright Futures: Promoting children and young people's mental health.* The Mental Health Foundation: London and Glasgow. www.mentalhealth.org.uk

Millward L.M., Morgan A., Kelly M.P. (2003) *Prevention and reduction of accidental injury in children and older people: Evidence Briefing.* Health Development Agency: London. www.hda.nhs.uk/evidence

Mitchell G. and Baptiste L. (3 February 2004) Developing links between school nursing and CAMHS. *Nursing Times* 100:5, 36-39.

Morrow V. (2001) *Networks and neighbourhoods: children's and young people's perspectives.* Health Development Agency: London. www.had-online.org.uk

Mitchell G., Baptiste L., Potel D. (3 February 2004) Developing links between school nursing and CAMHS. *Nursing Times* 100:5, 36-39.

MSF/CPHVA (2001) *Making the grade: grading guidance and the school nurse salary survey 2001.* MSF/CPHVA: London.

Mukherjee S., Lightfoot J., Sloper P. (2000) *Improving communication between health and education for children with chronic illness or physical disability.* NHS 1740 7.00 SM/JL/PS and Social Policy Research Unit, University of York: York.

Mukherjee S., Lightfoot J., Sloper P. (2002) Communicating about pupils in mainstream school with special health needs: the NHS perspective. *Child: Care & Development* 28:1, 21-27.

Mulvihill C. and Quigley R. (2003) *The Management of Obesity and Overweight: An Analysis of Reviews of Diet, Physical Activity and Behavioural Approaches.* Health Development Agency: London.

Naidoo J. and Wills J. (1998) *Health Promotion Foundations for Practice.* Bailliere Tindal: London.

Nash W., Thruston M., Baly M. (1985) *Health at School.* William Heinemann Medical Books: London.

National Assembly for Wales (2001a) *Improving Health in Wales: The future of primary care.* National Assembly for Wales: Cardiff.

National Assembly for Wales (2001b) *Improving Health in Wales: A Plan for the NHS with its partners.* National Assembly for Wales: Cardiff.

National Assembly for Wales (2001c) *Improving Health in Wales: structural change in the NHS in Wales.* National Assembly for Wales: Cardiff.

National Assembly for Wales (2001d) *Promoting health and well being: Implementing the national health promotion strategy.* National Assembly for Wales: Cardiff.

National Children's Bureau (1996) *Developing the role of the school nurse in sex education: Forum Factsheet 9.* National Children's Bureau: London.

National Clearing House on Child Abuse and Neglect Information and National Adoption Information Clearing House (2003) *Definitions of child abuse and neglect.* National Clearing House: London.

National Screening Committee – Royal College of Paediatrics and Child Health (1998) *Systematic reviews in child health. Report on a seminar entitled 'Evolution or Revolution'.* NHS Executive: London.

Nelson M. and Quinney D. (1997) Evaluating a school based health clinic. *Health visitor* 70:11, 419-421.

NHS Centre for Reviews and Dissemination (1997) *Preventing and reducing the adverse effects of unintended teenage pregnancies* 3:1.

NHS Centre for Reviews and Dissemination (2002) *The prevention and treatment of childhood obesity. Effective Health Care* 7: 6, 8.

NHS Education for Scotland (2004f) *Promoting the Wellbeing and Meeting the Mental Health Needs of Children and Young People: A Development Framework for Communities, Agencies and Specialists Involved in Supporting Children, Young People and Their Families*. www.qacpd.org.uk

NHS Executive (1995) *Developing NHS purchasing and GP fundholding: towards a primarycare-led NHS*. NHSE: Leeds.

NHS Executive (1999) *Public Health Practice Resource Pack*. NHS Eastern Region: London.

NHS Executive (October 2000) *School Nursing: Scoping Study – The Health Visitor and School Nurse Development Programme*. NHS Executive Northwest: London.

NHS Executive (April 2001) *Implementing the NHS Plan – Modern Matrons: Strengthening the role of ward sisters and introducing senior sisters*. Department of Health: London. www.doh.gov.uk/coinh.htm

NHS Health Advisory Service (1995) *Together we stand: child and adolescent mental health services*. The Stationery Office: London.

NHS Scotland (2004a) *Adventures in Foodland: Ideas for making food fun from an early age*. NHS Scotland: Edinburgh. www.ltscotland.org.uk/earlyyears/Foodland.asp

NHS Scotland (2004b) *Smoking Cessation Guidelines for Scotland: 2004 Update*. NHS Scotland and ASH Scotland. www.healthscotland.com/tobacco

NHS Scotland Immunisation Website – www.healthscotland.com/immunisation/

Northern Ireland Department of Health, Social Services and Public Safety (2000) *The Contribution of Nurses, Midwives & Health Visitors*. Working Paper No. 2. Northern Ireland Assembly: Belfast.

Northern Ireland Department of Health, Social Services and Public Safety (2000) *Investing for Health. A Consultation Paper*. Northern Ireland Assembly: Belfast.

Northern Ireland Department of Health, Social Services and Public Safety (February 2001) *A Nursing Vision of Public Health: All Ireland Statement on Public Health Nursing*. Northern Ireland Assembly: Belfast. www.dhsspsni.gov.uk/publications/archived/2001/nurse_vision.pdf

Northern Ireland Department of Health, Social Services and Public Safety (November 2002) *Teenage Pregnancy and Parenthood: Strategy & Action Plan 2002 - 2007*. Northern Ireland Assembly: Belfast. www.dhsspsni.gov.uk/publications/2003/teenage-pregnancy-action02-07.pdf

Northern Ireland Department of Health, Social Services and Public Safety (June 2003) *A Five Year Tobacco Action Plan: 2003 - 2008*. Northern Ireland Assembly: Belfast. www.dhsspsni.gov.uk/publications/2003/tobaccoplan.pdf

Northern Ireland Department of Health, Social Services and Public Safety (2003) *Drugs and Alcohol Campaign: A guide*. Northern Ireland Assembly: Belfast. www.dhsspsni.gov.uk/publications/2003/Drugalcohol.pdf

Northern Ireland Department of Health, Social Services and Public Safety (2003) *From Vision to Action – strengthening the nursing contribution to public health*. DHSSPS: Belfast.

Northern Ireland Department of Health, Social Services and Public Safety (November 2003) *Strategic Direction in Community Nursing in Northern Ireland: Position Paper*. Northern Ireland Assembly: Belfast. www.dhsspsni.gov.uk/publications/2004/strat_direction_comm_nursing_ni_nov03.pdf

Northern Ireland Department of Health, Social Services and Public Safety (June 2004) *A Five Year Physical Activity Strategy and Action Plan: Consultative Document*. Northern Ireland Assembly: Belfast. www.dhsspsni.gov.uk/publications/2004/physicalactivity/consult_document.pdf

Northern Ireland Department of Health, Social Services and Public Safety (December 2004) *A healthier future: A Twenty Year Vision for Health and Wellbeing in Northern Ireland 2005 - 2025*. Northern Ireland Assembly: Belfast. www.dhsspsni.gov.uk/publications/2004/healthyfuture-execsummary.pdf

Northern Ireland Department of Health, Social Services and Public Safety (June 2004) *A Five Year Physical Activity Strategy and Action Plan. Consultative Document*. DHSSPS: Belfast. www.dhsspsni.gov.uk/publications/2004/physicalactivity/consult_document.pdf

Northern Ireland Drug and Alcohol Strategy Team (2003) *Northern Ireland Drugs and Alcohol Campaign*. Department of Health, Social Services and Public Safety. Northern Ireland Assembly: Belfast. www.dhsspsni.gov.uk/publications/2003/Drugalcohol.pdf

Nursing and Midwifery Council (2002) *Code of Professional Conduct*. NMC: London.

Office for Standards in Education (2005) *Personal, social and health education in secondary schools*. www.ofsted.gov.uk

Olds D.L., Hill P.L., O'Brien R. (2003) Taking preventive intervention to scale: the nurse-family partnership. *Cognitive and behavioral practice* 10, 278-290.

Osborne N. (March 2000) Children's voices: evaluation of a school drop-in health clinic. *Community practitioner* 73:3, 516-518.

O'Toole A., O'Toole R., Webster S., Lucal B. (1997) Nurses' diagnostic work on possible physical child abuse. *Public Health Nursing* 14, 137-142.

Ovretveit J., Mathias P., Thompson T. (eds) (1997) *Interprofessional Working for Health and Social Care*. Macmillan Press: London.

Owen P. (2000) Public health – origins and definitions. *Journal of Community Nursing* 14:10, 13-14.

Owens P., Carrier J, Hodder J. (eds) (1995) *Interprofessional Issues in Community and Primary Health Care*. Macmillan Press: London.

Participation Education Group (PEG) in partnership with the Newcastle City health NHS Trust and Child Health Rights Action Group (1997) *School Can Seriously Damage Your Health: How Children Think School Affects and Deals with Their Health*. PEG: Newcastle.

Paavilainen E. and Astedt-Kurki P. (1997) The client-nurse relationship as experienced by public health nurses: toward better collaboration. *Public Health Nursing* 14, 137-142.

Paavilainen E., Astedt-Kurki P., Paunonen M. (2000) School nurses' operational modes and ways of collaborating in caring for child abusing families in Finland. *Journal of Clinical Nursing* 9, 742-750.

Pearce A., Finalay F., Bailey S. (March 1997) Parents' perceptions of routine school entry medicals. *Health visitor* 70:3, 101-102.

Peck E., Gulliver P., Towell D. (2002) Governance of partnership between health and social services: the experience in Somerset. *Health and Social Care in the Community* 10:5, 331-341.

Peckham S. and Carlson C. (2003) Bringing health care to schools. *Nursing Standard* 17:20, 33-38.

Pencheon D., Guest C., Melzer D., Muir Gray J.A. (eds) (2001) *Oxford Handbook of Public Health Practice*. Oxford University Press: Oxford.

Perkins E.R. (1989) The school health service through parents' eyes. *Archives of Disease in Childhood* 64, 1088-1091.

Petford C. and Howkins E. (1998) *Parenting programmes: Parents and professionals working together – Parenting project established by East Berkshire Community Trust*. University of Reading: Reading.

Polnay L. (Chair) (1995) *Health needs of school age children: Report of a Joint Working Party*. British Paediatric Association: London.

Polnay L. (1998) A school health service for children: a commentary. *Children & Society* 12:98, 100.

Poulton B., Mason C., McKenna H., Lynch C., Keeney S. (2000) *The Contribution of Nurses Midwives and Health Visitors to the Public Health Agenda*. Department of Health, Social Services and Public Safety: Northern Ireland.

Proctor S. (1998) Evaluation of nursing practice in schools. *Journal of School Health* 56:7, 272-275.

Richardson-Todd B. (October 2002) GPs: Do they know what school nurses do? *Primary Health Care* 12:8, 38-41.

Rafferty A.M., Traynor M., Thompson D.R., Ilott I., White E. (2003) Research in nursing, midwifery, and the allied health professions: quantum leap required for quality research. *British Medical Journal* 326, 833-834.

Reeve S. (January 2002) Sex education takes to the road. *Nursing Times* 98:05.

Richardson-Todd B. (2002) GPs: Do they know what school nurses do? *Primary Health Care* 12:8, 38-41.

Richardson-Todd B. (6 August 2003) Setting up a nurse-run young person's drop-in clinic. *Nursing Standard* 17:47, 38-41.

Roden D. (December 1997) Proving the value of school nursing services. *Health visitor* 70:12, 462-463.

Rogers E., Moon A., Mullee M. (1998) Developing the 'health promoting school' – a national survey of health schools awards. *Public Health* 112, 37-40.

Rogers L.L. (1908) Some Phases of School Nursing. *American Journal of Nursing* 8:12, 966-974. Reprinted (October 2002) *Journal of School Nursing* 18:5, 253-256. www.nasn.org/100year AJN LinaRogers.htm

Romano-Critchley G. and Somerville A. (2000) *Consent, rights and choices for children and young people*. British Medical Association: London.

Ross H.A. (2001) *Out Through the School Gates: A Review of School Nursing*. (unpublished) Tendring PCT: Essex.

Ross S. (1999) The clinical nurse specialist's role in school health. *Clinical Nurse Specialist* 13, 28-33.

Rote S. (1997) Losing sight of the future. *Nursing Times* 93:24, 58-59.

Royal College of General Practitioners, Royal College of Nursing (2002) *Getting it right for teenagers in your practice*. RCGP: London.

Ryberg J.W., Keller T., Hine B., Christeson E. (February 2003) Data Speak: Influencing School Health Policy Through Research. *The Journal of School Nursing* 19:1, 17-22.

Sackman T. (September 1998) Influencing the future. *Community Practitioner* 71:9, 281.

Sadler C. (August 1999) Building brighter futures. *Community Practitioner* 72:8, 246-247.

Sadler C. (June 2004) The fat of the land. *Nursing Standard* 18:41, 21-22.

Sadler J. (December 1999) Supporting children with special medical needs. *Community Practitioner* 72:12, 398-400.

Schonfield D.J. (1996) Talking with school-age children about AIDS and death. *Journal of School Nursing* 12, 26-32.

Schools Health Education Unit (April 2005) *Young People in 2004*. SHEU: Exeter.

Scottish Executive (1999a) *Learning Together – A Strategy for Education, Training and Lifelong Learning for all staff in the National Health Service in Scotland*. HMSO: Edinburgh. www.scotland.gov.uk/learningtogether/

Scottish Executive (1999b) *Making it Work Together – A programme for government*. HMSO: Edinburgh. www.scotland.gov.uk/library2/doc03/miwt-00.htm

Scottish Executive (1999c) *Social Justice – A Scotland where EVERYONE matters*. HMSO: Edinburgh. www.scotland.gov.uk/library2/doc07/sjmd-00.htm

Scottish Executive (1999d) *The Review of the Public Health Function in Scotland*. HMSO: Edinburgh. www.scotland.gov.uk/cru/resfinds/grf04-00.htm

Scottish Executive (1999e) *Towards a Healthier Scotland*. Scottish Executive: Edinburgh. (Announced the establishment of four locally based health demonstration projects in priority areas of child health, the sexual health of young people, coronary heart disease and cancer, to act as testing grounds for action and a learning resource for the rest of Scotland.) www.scotland.gov.uk/library/documents-w7/tahs-00.htm

Scottish Executive (2000a) *Chief Medical Officer's Report – Health in Scotland 1999*. HMSO: Edinburgh.

Scottish Executive (2000b) *Community Care: A Joint Future*. HMSO: Edinburgh.

Scottish Executive (2000c) *Fair Shares for All – the Report of the National Review of Resource allocation for the NHS in Scotland*. HMSO: Edinburgh.

Scottish Executive (2000e) *Our National Health – A Plan for Action, a Plan for Change*. HMSO: Edinburgh. www.scotland.gov.uk/library3/health/onh-00.asp

Scottish Executive (2000f) *Protecting Children – A Shared Responsibility*. HMSO: Edinburgh. www.scotland.gov.uk/library2/doc11/pcsr-00.asp

Scottish Executive (2000g) *Report of the Working Group on Sex Education in Scottish Schools*. Scottish Executive: Edinburgh. www.scotland.gov.uk/library2/doc16/sexedwg.pdf

Scottish Executive (2001a) *Caring for Scotland: The Strategy for Nursing and Midwifery in Scotland*. HMSO: Edinburgh. www.scotland.gov.uk/library3/health/snms-00.asp

Scottish Executive (2001b) *For Scotland's Children – Better Integrated Children's Services*. Scottish Executive: Edinburgh. www.scotland.gov.uk/library3/education/fcsr-00.asp

Scottish Executive (2001c) *Nursing for Health. The Effectiveness of Public Health Nursing: A Review of Systematic Reviews*. Scottish Executive: Edinburgh.

Scottish Executive (2001d) *Nursing for Health – A Review of the Contribution of Nurses, Midwives and Health Visitors to Improving the Public's Health in Scotland*. Scottish Executive: Edinburgh. www.scotland.go.uk/library3/health/ehpnr-00.asp

Scottish Executive (2001e) *Patient Focus and Public Involvement*. Scottish Executive: Edinburgh. www.scotland.gov.uk/library3/health/pfpi.pdf

Scottish Executive (2002a) *Growing Support: A Review of Services for Vulnerable Families with Very Young Children*. Scottish Executive: Edinburgh. www.scotland.gov.uk/library5/social/gsrs.pdf

Scottish Executive (2002b) *Hungry for Success: A Whole School Approach to School Meals in Scotland*. Scottish Executive: Edinburgh. www.scotland.gov.uk/library5/ education/hfs.pdf

Scottish Executive (2002c) *It's Everyone's Job to Make Sure I'm Alright: Report of the Child Protection Audit and Review*. Scottish Executive: Edinburgh. www.scotland.gov.uk/library5/education/iaar-03.asp

Scottish Executive (2003a) *A Scottish Framework for Nursing in Schools*. Scottish Executive: Edinburgh. www.scotland.gov.uk/library5/education/sfns-00.asp

Scottish Executive (2003b) *Getting our Priorities Right – Good Practice for Working with Children and Families Affected by Substance Misuse*. Scottish Executive: Edinburgh. www.scotland.gov.uk/library5/education/gopr.pdf

Scottish Executive (2003c) *Improving Health in Scotland – The Challenge*. Scottish Executive: Edinburgh. www.scotland.gov.uk/library5/health/ihis-00.asp

Scottish Executive (2003d) *Responding to Domestic Abuse: Guidelines for Health Care Workers in NHS Scotland*. Scottish Executive: Edinburgh. www.scotland.gov.uk/library5/health/rdag-00.asp

Scottish Executive (2003e) *Sharing Information About Children At Risk: A Guide to Good Practice*. Scottish Executive: Edinburgh. www.scotland.gov.uk/library5/health/sicr-00.asp

Scottish Executive (2004a) *A Breath of Fresh Air for Scotland*. Scottish Executive: Edinburgh. www.scotland.gov.uk/library5/health/abfa.pdf

Scottish Executive (2004b) *Children and Young People's Mental Health: A Draft Framework for Promotion, Prevention and Care*. Scottish Executive: Edinburgh. www.scotland.gov.uk/consultations/health/cypmh-00.asp

Scottish Executive (2004c) *Community Health Partnerships and Integrated Children's Services*. Scottish Executive: Edinburgh. www.show.scot.nhs.uk/sehd/chp/Pages/advicenotes.htm

Scottish Executive (2004d) *Community Health Partnerships: Statutory Guidance*. Scottish Executive: Edinburgh. www.show.scot.nhs.uk/sehd/chp/Pages/CHPfinal%20guidanceOCT2.pdf

Scottish Executive (2004e) *Education (Additional Support for Learning) (Scotland) Act 2004*. Scottish Executive: Edinburgh. www.scotland.gov.uk/Topics/Education/School-Education/19094/17176

Scottish Executive (2004f) *Getting It Right For Every Child: Summary Report on the Responses to the Phase One Consultation on the Review of the Children's Hearing System*. Scottish Executive: Edinburgh. www.scotland.gov.uk/library5/education/girsum.pdf

Scottish Executive (2004g) *Hidden Harm: Scottish Executive Response to the Report of the Inquiry by the Advisory Council on the Misuse of Drugs*. Scottish Executive: Edinburgh. www.scotland.gov.uk/library5/health/hhser.pdf

Scottish Executive (2004h) *Protecting Children and Young People: A Framework for Standards*. Scottish Executive: Edinburgh. www.scotland.gov.uk/about/ED/CnF/00017834/page1423929284.pdf

Scottish Executive (2004i) *Protecting Children and Young People: The Charter.* Scottish Executive: Edinburgh. www.scotland.gov.uk/library5/education/ccel.pdf

Scottish Executive (2004j) *Sharing Information About Children At Risk: A Guide to Good Practice.* Scottish Executive: Edinburgh. www.show.scot.nhs.uk/sehd/cmo/ CMO(2004)19.pdf

Scottish Executive (2004k) *Towards Oral Health in Children – A Consultation Document on Children's Oral Health in Scotland.* Scottish Executive: Edinburgh. www.scotland.gov.uk/ consultations/health/ccoh.pdf

Scottish Executive (2005a) *Health for all children 4: Guidance on Implementation in Scotland.* Scottish Executive: Edinburgh. www.scotland.gov.uk/consultations/health/hfac-00.asp

Scottish Executive (2005b) *Respect and Responsibility – Strategy and Action Plan for Improving Sexual Health.* Scottish Executive: Edinburgh. www.scotland.gov.uk/library5/health/ shsf.pdf

Scottish Executive (to be published) *Integrated Assessment Framework for Scotland's Children.* Scottish Executive: Edinburgh.

Scottish Executive (planned for 2007, 2008, and 2009) *Growing Up in Scotland.* Longitudinal social survey to monitor the impact of Scottish Executive early years policies on longer term outcomes for children and young people by tracking a number of representative cohorts of children from birth until the age of 5. The first cross-sectional times series data are expected to be available for 2-3 year olds in 2007, 3-4 years olds in 2008 and 4-5 year olds in 2009. Scottish Executive: Edinburgh.

Scottish Executive Social Research (2005) *Health for all Children Draft Guidance on Implementation in Scotland: Analysis of Consultation Responses.* Scottish Executive: Edinburgh.

Scottish Executive Policy Unit (2000) *Youth Crime in Scotland.* HMSO: Edinburgh.

Scottish Health Promoting Schools Unit (2004) *Being Well – Doing Well: A Framework for Health Promoting Schools in Scotland.* Scottish Executive: Edinburgh. www.ltscotland.org.uk/wholeschoolissues/files/ beingwelldoingwell.pdf

Scottish Office (1996a) *Health services in schools – report of a policy review.* HMSO: Edinburgh.

Scottish Office (1996b) *Choice and Opportunity – Primary Care: The Future.* Department of Health. London and The Scottish Office: Edinburgh.

Scottish Office (1997) *Scotland's Children: The Children (Scotland) Act 1995 Regulations and Guidance – Volume 1: Support and Protection for Children and Their Families.* Scottish Office: Edinburgh.

Scottish Office (1998a) *Designed to Care – Reviewing the National Health Service in Scotland.* HMSO: Edinburgh.

Scottish Office (1998b) *New Community Schools Prospectus.* Crown Copyright.

Scottish Office (1999) *Towards a Healthier Scotland – A White Paper on Health.* HMSO: Norwich.

Scottish Office Central Research Unit (1999) *Supporting Parenting in Scotland – a mapping exercise.* HMSO: Edinburgh.

Scowen P. (1997) Meeting the health needs of the school-aged child: HVA Centenary Conference 1996 report. *Professional Care of Mother & Child.* 7:1, 5-6.

Scriven A. and Orme J. (eds) (2001,2nd ed) *Health Promotion, Professional Perspectives.* Palgrave in association with The Open University: Hampshire.

Seedhouse D. (2002) Commitment to health: a shared ethical bond between professions. *Journal of Interprofessional Care* 16:3, 249-260.

Selby M. (1999) The doctor who changed my view. How to drive away teenagers. *British Medical Journal* 318, 1323.

Sharples A., Gibson S., Galvin K. (2002) 'Floating support': implications for interprofessional working. *Journal of Interprofessional Care* 16:4, 311-312.

Sheetz A.H. (2003) Developing School Health Services in Massachusetts: A Public Health Model. *The Journal of School Nursing* 19:4, 204-211.

Shepherd J., Stuart D. (May 2001) School nurse health interviews: effectiveness and alternatives. *Community Practitioner* 74:5, 185-189.

Short R.V. (July 2004) Teaching safe sex in English schools. *The Lancet* 364:9431, 307-308.

Siminerio L.M. and Koerbel G. (September 2000) A diabetes education programme for school personnel. *Practical Diabetes International* 17:6, 174-177.

Slack P.A. (1978) *School Nursing.* Balliere Tindall: London.

Smith G.C., Powell A., Reynolds K., Campbell C.A. (1990) The five year school medical – time for change. *Archives of Disease in Childhood* 65:2, 225-227.

Smith G. (March 2003) Emergency contraception: a pilot study by school nurses. *Nursing Times* 99:12.

Social Exclusion Unit (1999) *Teenage Pregnancy.* HMSO: Norwich.

Social Services Inspectorate (2002) *Modern Social Services: A commitment to the future. The 12th Annual Report of the Chief Inspector of Social Services.* Department of Health: London.

St Leger (1999) The opportunities and effectiveness of the health promoting primary school in improving child health – a review of the claims and evidence. *Health Education Research* 14:1, p 51 (20 pages on-line). her.oupjournals.org/cgi/ content/full/14/1/51?maxtoshow=&HITS=10&hits=10&RES

Starfield B. (September/October 2004) U.S. Child Health: What's Amiss, And What Should Be Done About It? *Health Affairs* 23:5, 165-170.

Steen J. (May 1997) "A strategy for school nursing". *Health visitor* 70:05, 101.

Stephenson J.M., Strange V., Forrest S., Oakley A., Copas A., Allen E., Babiker A., Black S., Ali M., Monterio H., Johnson A.M. (2004) Pupil-led sex education in England (RIPPLE study): cluster-randomised intervention trial. *The Lancet* 364, 338-346.

Stevens A. and Raftery J. (eds.) (1997) *Health Care Needs Assessment: The epidiologically based needs assessment review.* Radcliffe Medical Press: Oxford and New York.

Strenlow M.S. (1987) *Nursing in Educational Settings.* Harper Row Ltd: London.

Sutton H. (2001) Sexual Health Promotion: Reducing the Rate of Teenage Pregnancy. *Paediatric Nursing* 13:3, 33-37.

Sutton S., Gill J., Millard L. (16 June 2004) Reshaping a school health nursing service. *Nursing Standard* 18:40, 33-35.

Svenson G.R. (1998) *Annotated Bibliography about Youth AIDS Peer Education in Europe.* European Commission: Lund.

Swinkels A., Albarran J.W., Means R.I., Mitchell T., Stewart M.C. (2002) Evidence-based practice in health and social care: where are we now? *Journal of Interprofessional Care* 16:4, 335-347.

Symonds A. and Kelly A. (eds) (1998) *The Social Construct of Community Care.* Macmillan: Basingstoke.

Thies K. (December 1999) Identifying the educational implications of chronic illness in school children. *Journal of School Health* 69:10, 392-397.

Thistle S. (2003) *Secondary schools and sexual health services.* Sex Education Forum: London.

Thistle S. and Ray C. (2002) Sex and relationships education: the role of the school nurse. *Nursing Standard* 17:1, 44-55.

Thompson M., Coll X., Wilkinson S. Uitenbroek D., Tobias A. (2003) Evaluation of a Mental Health Service for Young Children: Development, Outcome and Satisfaction. *Child and Adolescent Mental Health* 8:2, 68-77.

Thurtle V. (1997) Lessons from the past. *Primary Health Care* 7, 15-16.

Thurtle V. (2001) School Nursing In Sines D. (ed.) *Community Healthcare Nursing.* Blackwell Science: London.

Todd R. (2003) Serving up a nurse-run young person's drop-in clinic. *Nursing Standard* 17:47, 38-41.

Torevell H. (2000) *Routine child health interviews for children age eight and nine years: Are they an effective use of school nursing time?* Unpublished dissertation for Master of Public Health. Nuffield Institute of Health, University of Leeds: Leeds.

Tumin W. (2001) *Independent Advisory Group on Teenage Pregnancy: First Annual Report.* Department of Health: London.

Turner J. and Lazenbatt A. (July 2003) *Community Health Nursing: Current Practice and Possible Futures.* Nursing, Midwifery and Advisory Group, Department of Health, Social Services and Public Safety: Belfast. www.dhsspsni.gov.uk/publications/2004/community_Health_Nursing.pdf

Turner T. (August 1999) Promoting public health. *Community Practitioner* 72:8, 238-240.

Turtle J., Jones A., Hickman M. (1997) *Young people and health: the health behaviour of school-aged children – Summary of key findings.* Health Education Authority: London.

UK Parliament (2004) *Children Act.* HMSO: Norwich. www.hmso.gov.uk/acts/acts2004/20040031.htm

UNICEF (2005) *Child Poverty in Rich Countries 2005: Innocenti Report Card No. 6.* Innocenti Research Centre, UNICEF: Florence Italy.

United Nations (1989) *United Nations Convention on the Rights of the Child .* UN: Geneva.

United Nations (1992) *Conventions on the Rights of the Child,* Treaty Series 44. HMSO: Norwich.

United Nations International Children's Emergency Fund (2002) *The State of the World's Children.* UNICEF: New York.

University of East Anglia in association with the National Children's Bureau (September 2005) *Realising children's trust arrangements: National Evaluation of Children's Trusts. Phase 1 Report.*

Vernon S. (May 2003) Toilet facilities in schools. *Nursing Times* 99:19.

Wainwright P., Thomas J., Jones M. (2000) Health promotion and the role of the school nurse: a systematic reveiw. *Journal of Advanced Nursing* 32:5, 1083-1091.

Wales M. (1941) *The Public Health Nurse in Action.* Macmillan Publishing Company: New York.

Walker Z.A.K., Townsend J.L. (1999) The role of general practice in promoting teenage health: A review of the literature. *Family Practice* 16, 164-172.

Walker Z.A.K., Townsend J.L., Bell J., Marshall S. (1999) An opportunity for teenage health promotion in general practice: an assessment of current provision and needs. *Health Education Journal* 58, 218-227.

Wallis L. (November 1999) Monsters under the bed. *Nursing Standard* 14:7, 18-19.

Ward H., Holmes L., Moyers S., Munro E.R., Poursanidou K. (2004) *Safeguarding children: a scoping study of research in three areas.* Centre for Child and Family Research: Loughborough.

Waterhouse R. (2000) *Lost in Care: The Report of the Tribunal of Inquiry into the abuse of children in care in the former county council areas of Gwynedd and Clwyd since 1974.* HC201: Cardiff.

Watters M. (February 1999) *Providing Health services to School Children: A Literature Review of the School Nursing Service.* Public Health Research and Resource Centre: University of Salford.

Webber I. (1998) Professions and School Nursing. In Symonds A. and Kelly A. (eds) *The Social Construct of Community Care.* Macmillan: Basingstoke.

Webster C. and French J. (2002) The Cycle of Conflict: The History of the Public Health. In Adams A., Amos L., Munro J. (eds) *Promoting Health: Politics and Practice.* Sage Publications: London.

Webster D. (March 1999) *The School Nurse Role in Healthy School Schemes.* Mancunian Health Promotion: Manchester.

Welford H. (August 1999) Food for thought. *Community Practitioner* 72:8, 241-242.

Wellings K., Nanchahal K., Macdowall W., McManus S., Erens B., Mercer C.H., Johnson A.M., Copas A.J., Korovessis C., Fenton K.A., Field J. (1 December 2001) Sexual Behaviour in Britain: early heterosexual experience. *The Lancet* 358:9296, 1843-1850.

Wellings K., Wadsworth J., Johnson A.M., Field J., Whitaker I., Field B. (12 August 1995) Provision of sex education and early sexual experience: the relation examined. *British Medical Journal* 311, 417-420.

Welsh Assembly Government (2004a) *Children and Young People: Rights to action.* Welsh National Assembly: Cardiff. www.wales.gov.uk/subichildren/content/consultations/cyp04-cover-e.pdf

Welsh Assembly Government (2004b) *The National Service Framework for children, young people and maternity services in Wales.* Welsh National Assembly: Cardiff.

Welsh Assembly Government (April 2004c) *Report of the Child Poverty Task Group.* Welsh National Assembly: Cardiff. www.wales.gov.uk/organicabinet/SubCmt-eeMeetings/children/papers/cyp(03-04)30annex.pdf

Welsh Assembly Government (February 2005) *A Fair Future for Our Children: The Strategy of the Welsh Assembly Government for Tackling Child Poverty.* Welsh National Assembly: Cardiff. www.wales.gov.uk/subichildren/content/summary-action-plan-e.pdf

Welsh Assembly Government (March 2005) *Parenting Action Plan: Supporting mothers, fathers and carers with raising children in Wales Draft for Consultation.* Welsh National Assembly: Cardiff. www.wales.gov.uk/subichildren/ content/consultations/pap-summary-e.pdf

Welsh Office (1997) *Supporting Pupils with Medical Needs in Schools.* Welsh Office Circular 34/37, Welsh Health Circular 97/31, Welsh Office Education Department: Cardiff.

Wheatley M. (1998) Running a teenage 'drop-in' in school. *Primary Health Care* 8:3, 26-29.

Whetton T. and Jackson P. (December 1996) A school needs weighting formula. *Primary Health Care* 6:11, 14-15.

While A. and Bamunoba M. (1992) School nursing children's contract with the school health service. *Health visitor* 65:2, 53-54.

While A.E. and Barriball K.L. (1993) School nursing: history, present practice and possibilities reviewed. *Journal of Advanced Nursing* 20, 324-330.

Whitehead D. (2001) A social cognitive model for health education/health promotion practice. *Journal of Advanced Nursing* 36:3, 417-425.

Whitmarsh J. (26 March 1997) School nurses' skills in sexual health education. *Nursing Standard* 11:27, 35-41.

Whitmore K. and Bax M.C.O. (1990) Checking the health of school entrants. *Archives of Disease in Childhood* 65, 320-326.

Wicklander M.K. (June 2005) The United Kingdom National Healthy School Standard: A Framework for Strengthening the School Nurse Role. *The Journal of School Nursing* 21:3, 132-138.

Williams N.S. (1998) Routine versus selective school nurse entrant medical – a retrospective study on the Isle of Man. *Public Health* 112:1, 41-46.

Wold S.J. (1981) *School Nursing: A Framework for Practice.* Reprinted by Sunrise River Press: Minnesota USA.

Wolfe L.C. and Hootman J. (2003) The Role of the School Nurse in Providing School Health Services. *The Journal of School Nursing* 19:3, 127-129.

Woodcock C., Glickman M., Barker M., Power C. (1993) *Children, teenagers and health.* Open University Press: Buckingham.

World Health Organisation (1986) *Ottawa Charter for Health Promotion: The move towards a new public health.* WHO: Geneva.

World Health Organisation (1998) *Health 21 — Health for all in the 21st Century.* WHO: Copenhagen.

World Health Organisation (2000a) *The Family Nurse: Context, Conceptual Framework and Curriculum.* WHO: Geneva.

World Health Organisation (2000b) *Global Advisory Group on Nursing and Midwifery.* WHO: Geneva.

World Health Organisation (2000c) *Health Behaviour in School-aged Children: The Health of Youth.* WHO: Copenhagen. www.who.dk/

World Health Organisation (2000d) *Health Care Reforms: The Nursing Response.* WHO: Copenhagen.

World Health Organisation (2000e) *Munich Declaration. Nurses and Midwives: a Force for Health.* WHO: Copenhagen. EUR/00/50193096/6. www.who.int/health-services delivery/nursing/gagnm/index.htm

World Health Organisation (from 2000f) *The school health component of the Mega Country Health Promotion Network.* WHO: Geneva. www.who.int/entity/school_youth_health/mega/en/

World Health Organisation (from 2001a) *Global school health initiative*. WHO: Geneva. www.who.int/school_youth_health/gshi/en/

World Health Organisation (2001b) *Strengthening nursing and midwifery: Progress and Future Directions*. WHO: Geneva.

World Health Organisation (2001c) *Workshop on global health workforce strategy. Annecy France 9-12 December 2000*. WHO: Geneva.

World Health Organisation (2001d) *Workshop on Global Health Workforce Strategy: Final Report, Documents Summary*. WHO: Geneva.

Wylie I., Griffiths S., Junter D.J. (1999) Everywhere and nowhere – a Socratic dialogue on the new public health. *British Medical Journal* 319, 839-840.

Yamey G. (20 November 1999) Sexual and reproductive health: what about boys and men? *British Medical Journal* 319, 1315-1316.

Young B. and Arnold-Dean W. (Revised edition 2004) *Personal, social and health education (PSHE) certification programme for community nurses*. Department for Education and Skillls, Teenage Pregnancy Unit, and National Healthy School Programme by the Department of Health: London.